'Filled with humour, facts, and u
created a necessary and diges
and everyone who is mystified by, or just wants to kn
more about vaginas, and everything that goes with them.'

TANYA REYNOLDS

'I love love love this book. It is such an important read that it should be given to every woman in the world so that they can understand and celebrate the superpower that is their womanhood.'

ANDREA MCLEAN

'Your vagina now has an owner's manual and it's about time! This book is for any vulva owner who has wanted more pleasure, less shame and a roadmap for accepting and understanding their body.'

EMILY MORSE, DOCTOR OF HUMAN SEXUALITY, HOST OF SEX WITH EMILY PODCAST

THE HAPPY VAGINA

Pavilion
An imprint of HarperCollinsPublishers Ltd
1 London Bridge Street
London SE1 9GF

www.harpercollins.co.uk

HarperCollinsPublishers
1st Floor, Watermarque Building
Ringsend Road Dublin 4
Ireland

10 9 8 7 6 5 4 3 2 1

First published in Great Britain by Pavilion, an imprint of HarperCollinsPublishers Ltd 2022

 A catalogue record for this book is available from the British Library.

ISBN 978-1-911663-85-0

Reproduction by Rival Colour Ltd., UK
Printed and bound by Toppan Leefung Ltd., China

Illustrator: Maja Tomljanovic

DISCLAIMERS:

This book is about vaginas and is for anyone who wants to know more about gynaecological, reproductive and sexual health.

The information in this book is true to the best of our knowledge. Any recommendations are made without guarantee on the part of the author or Pavilion Books. The author and publishers disclaim any liability in connection with this information.

This book is produced from independently certified FSC™ paper to ensure responsible forest management. For more information visit: www.harpercollins.co.uk/green

MIKA SIMMONS

THE HAPPY VAGINA

PAVILION

FOR ILIA AND ARIANNA

CONTENTS

MY STORY 6

GODDESS VIBES 8

CHAPTER 1

HYSTERICAL HISTRIONICS 10

CHAPTER 2

YOUR BODY, YOUR RESPONSIBILITY 30

CHAPTER 3

ANYTHING YOU CAN DO, I CAN DO BLEEDING 54

CHAPTER 4

THE SEX WAS SO GOOD, EVEN THE NEIGHBOURS HAD A CIGARETTE 78

CHAPTER 5

BE YOURSELF, EVERYONE ELSE IS TAKEN 106

BOOKS TO READ 124

INDEX 126

SPECIAL THANK YOUS 128

MY STORY

I became an activist in the female health space by accident really, after losing my mother, Rosie, aged just 54, to ovarian cancer.

For a long time, I struggled to understand why she had been taken from us so young and by this, the most brutal of female cancers. Hadn't she been a nurse, a carer, and a leader in the second wave of feminism, fighting for women's equality? It didn't make any sense.

Eventually, to heal and continue her legacy of protest, I began to dedicate my spare time and energy to campaigning for change in women's health. Through the work of my charity, Lady Garden Foundation, I wanted to help find better treatments for female cancers. And my podcast, The Happy Vagina, is about empowering women, through frank and intimate conversations, to know their bodies, demand better from health services and close not just the gender gap, but the pleasure gap too.

While on this journey, it has become increasingly apparent to me that, if there is one thing throughout history that has been wronged as much as it has been worshipped, it is women's bodies. Medicine, politics, religion, and social conditioning have all had a thoroughly improper and exaggerated influence on women's being – with many of the falsehoods told still negatively impacting us.

My intention with this book is to re-educate us all by shining a light on these ridiculous, historical myths and then debunk them by sharing the most unique, incredible and empowering facts about everything VAGINA, thereby encouraging a more open dialogue for everyone. And I do mean everyone – this book is about those who identify as women but all humans are welcome here. Because in order for deep change to happen, we have to take everyone with us. I hope this book will be just as enlightening for the woman who never had an orgasm as for the young men who are determined to be the best partner, or the Dad with teenage daughters who are fast becoming women. Everyone is invited.

The hardest part of this project was choosing what to put in – because both the misinformation about women's health, the missing stories and amazing facts are endless. At times, this felt overwhelming and so, in the end, I have simply chosen my favourites, hoping that you will be inspired by them too. If the content here sparks your interest or ignites your desire and you want to delve deeper, I have included a resources and further reading section at the back of the book, full of trailblazing women who inspire me.

I am not a historian or a women's health expert. I am simply a disobedient woman who has been acutely impacted by the gender health gap and who believes that women deserve to know the truth, so we can feel exceptional in and about ourselves... as the goddesses we truly are.

Love, Mika

PS If you don't like swearing, this book is not for you.

GODDESS VIBES

Before we start, let's get something straight – you are a goddess. Yes, that's right – I'm talking to YOU! You are a goddess.

You might not feel like a goddess, but you are one. Because the female body is amazing, complicated and divine, with supernatural powers from our immensely strong immune systems to a uterus that has the ability to crush a soda can. As such, at The Happy Vagina, we believe it should be fundamentally, thoroughly and eternally worshipped.

But before embarking on this inspirational and enlightening journey of goddess discovery together, we must first take a brief moment to go back, right back, to the very beginnings of modern medicine, to give you a little perspective on why, today, you might not feel like a goddess at all...

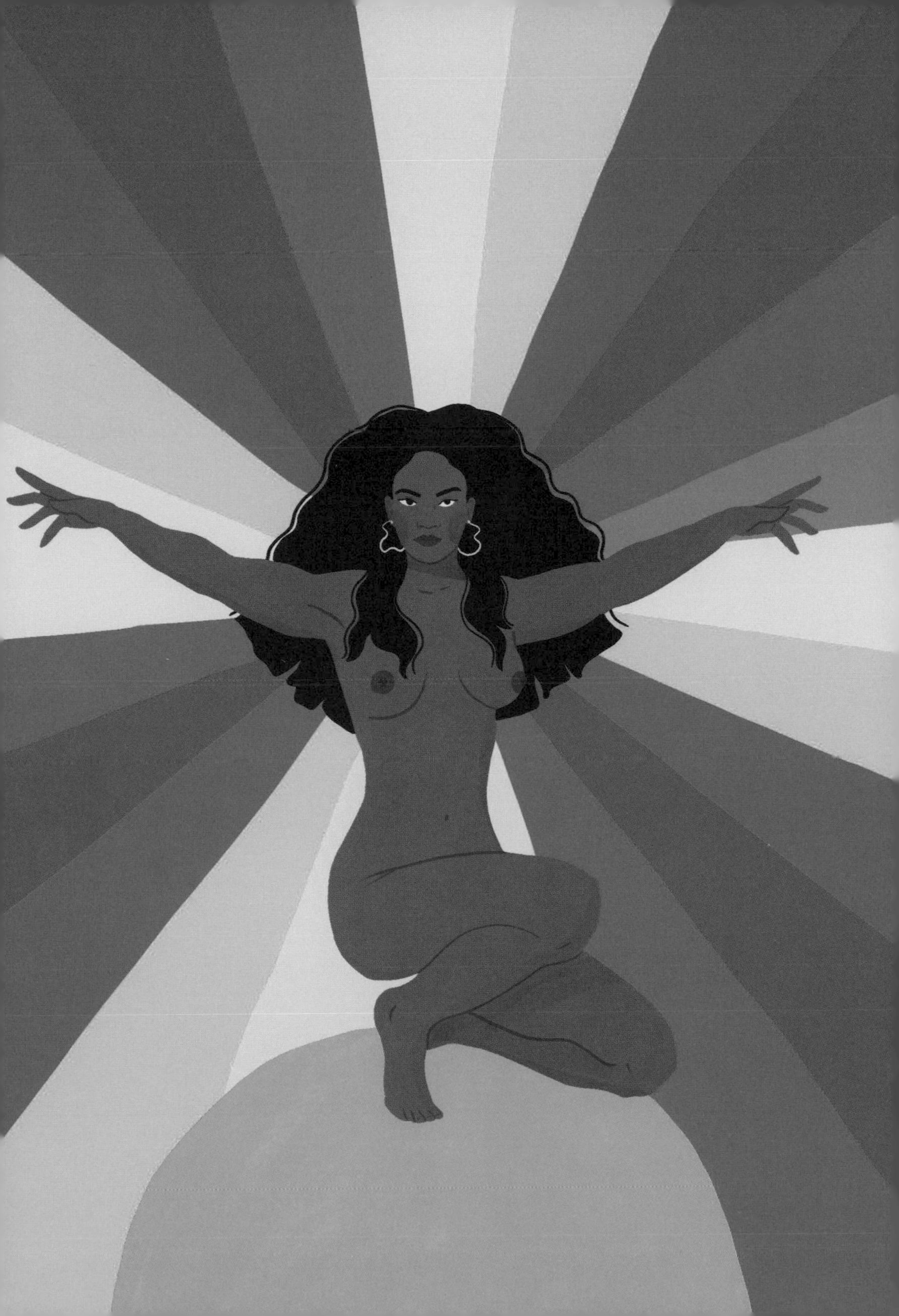

CHAPTER 1

HYSTERICAL HISTRIONICS

A POTTED HISTORY OF WOMEN'S HEALTH

THE ANCIENT GREEKS HAVE A LOT TO ANSWER FOR...

When it comes to modern medicine, the male body has long been assumed to be the 'better model', but it hasn't always been this way.

Women, women's bodies and even women's vaginas used to be worshipped as the epitome of anatomical design. Valued in their role as life givers and protectors of the earth, women were held as at least equal to men, if not superior. Almost every ancient culture has examples of maternal deities which honour the cycle of life – sexual union, birth, nurture and female creativity (see page 21).

So, where did it all go so wrong? To fully comprehend how all the sexist nonsense started, we have to look back at the often great, yet frequently deluded, philosophers of Ancient Greece. Although Greek philosophers didn't exactly invent misogyny, they did put forward the ridiculous suggestion that men were superior to women and should be dominant in the name of 'divine good'.

Whose divine good?
Theirs, obviously.

It almost certainly all started with a chap called Aristotle (c. 384–322 BC), who is sometimes described as the 'godfather of evidence-based medicine'.

It was this Aristotle (who, by the way, was not a doctor at all but simply a man who thought a lot) who made the biological assumption that the anatomy and physiology of the male form was the fully developed human, therefore concluding that a woman, by comparison, must be a 'deformed male'.

THE FIRST PROBLEM
FOR ALL OF US,
MEN AND WOMEN,
IS NOT TO LEARN,
BUT TO UNLEARN.

GLORIA STEINEM

AND WHAT, YOU MAY ASK, MAKES A WOMAN A 'PHYSICALLY FAULTY' HUMAN?

Why, her inability to produce semen, of course! Which, according to Aristotle, was the only thing necessary for human conception. In Aristotle's mind, woman was dormant in the act of procreation, simply an empty receptacle where 'glorious Man' could create a new human. **WTF?**

These Ancient Greek myths, featuring women as the inferior sex, then became the bedrock on which physicians developed a medical system that has pretty much wreaked havoc on women's health ever since.

First, there was the physician Hippocrates (c. 460–375 BC). Yes, the same Hippocrates of the medical world's Hippocratic oath. It was Hippocrates who was the first to use the term 'female hysteria' and claim that the cause of this disease lay in the 'abnormal movements' of the uterus in a woman's body.

Then there was Aretaeus (second century AD), who also believed that a woman's uterus wandered about her body like an 'animal within an animal', causing illness as it banged into the spleen or liver. What's more, he was convinced that these wandering wombs were attracted to fragrant smells and that, therefore, a physician could lure them back into place by presenting the vagina with pleasant scents. Hysterical!

Next up was the so-called creator of modern medicine, Galen (c. AD 131–210), who incidentally performed all his medical investigations on male animals.

While Galen made some progress by rejecting Aretaeus's myth of the wandering uterus – phew! – he sadly did far more damage when he claimed that a woman's reproductive organs were simply those of an 'underdeveloped male'.

Yes, that is correct, Galen firmly believed that the human body was basically unisexual and the two sexes were inside-out versions of each other, with the male of course being primary and the female secondary. It was also Galen who was responsible for the absurd idea that, like men, women produced an essential 'seed' that was necessary to procreate and released only upon orgasm.

As studies have consistently suggested that men experience orgasms during intercourse over 99% of the time, while in women, this occurs only around 50% – can you imagine the pressure?!

INVISIBLE WOMEN

But what happened next was, perhaps, worse than all of the Ancient Greeks' hypothesizing. In the early sixteenth century, the ban on the dissection of human corpses was finally lifted but as the practice was only permitted on hanged felons, the bodies were predominantly male. In fact, historians have found that male bodies were dissected two or three times as often as female bodies.

The consequences were devastating. Female reproductive and gynaecological anatomy was largely excluded from medical literature and, shockingly, it means they are still often misinterpreted today. For example, rarely do modern anatomical texts illustrate the clitoris in its full glory with 'legs' that extend deep inside the vaginal wall; the labia are commonly misrepresented as symmetrical and the vaginal canal is drawn as a huge gaping hole when, in fact, in its relaxed state the walls touch. More on that later (see page 39) but for now, back to the early sixteenth century and over to Italy.

In comes the legend that is Leonardo da Vinci (1452–1519). Have you ever noticed that, in his revered human anatomy sketches, the uteruses look more like those of other animals? Well, you'd be right. While Leonardo is famous for his meticulous observations of the human form, with many of his beautiful illustrations still relevant today, he fell somewhat short of accurate when sketching the female reproductive tract. Due to the difficulty of getting female bodies to study, Leonardo felt he had no choice but to fill in the gaps in his knowledge... with animal dissections!

Finally, and providing the last piece of the puzzle that set the stage for the gender health gap, there was Andreas Vesalius (1514–1564), considered the father of anatomy for his 1543 book *On the Fabric of the Human Body*. Vesalius not only prolonged the myth that the vagina was the female equivalent of the penis, he added in the catastrophic idea that the clitoris was an 'abnormal' part that didn't occur in healthy women and only existed in hermaphrodites. As if that wasn't enough, he also drew vessels between the vagina and breasts to demonstrate his belief that menstrual blood became milk. **Baffling!**

These patriarchal theories on human anatomy went on to dominate and influence medical science for the next 1,500 years.

RELIGION ALSO HAS A LOT TO ANSWER FOR

When women's bodies were finally freely dissected in the nineteenth century, images of reproductive systems were considered to be sinful and scandalous. So, most books either hid the images of genitals under flaps of paper, or omitted them entirely. University of Cambridge researchers recently discovered an anatomy book with a triangular cut out where the vagina would have appeared.

Don't even get us started on the incomprehensibly detrimental impact it had on women's sex lives and pleasure.

AN ACTUAL, REAL-LIFE VAGINA

It wasn't until the nineteenth century that a doctor finally got a good look inside a living vagina. Of course – it was a male doctor. But did he treat it with the respect and adoration it deserved? Of course not!

In the 1840s, James Marion Sims was a young Alabama doctor, who not only invented the vaginal speculum, which gynaecologists still use to open and see inside the vagina, he also pioneered the first surgery to repair vesicovaginal fistula (a complication of childbirth in which a hole opens between the vagina and the bladder). While Sims' innovations might have been considered breakthroughs, his methods were deeply unethical; experimenting on enslaved African American women, without anaesthesia, at a time when it would have been impossible for them to refuse. In April 2018, a statue of Sims in New York City's Central Park was taken down, to be replaced by a plaque that will give the names of the three women who Sims experimented upon: Betsey, Anarcha and Lucy.

THE HYSTERICAL IS HISTORICAL

Without any scientifically proven evidence, early medics, who were of course all men, took it upon themselves to construct a whole heap of nonsense to explain women's health conditions. Perhaps the one that has had the longest-lasting impact was the claim that pretty much any woman's health issue was due to something called 'hysteria'.

Hysteria? Yes, exactly that – hysteria! Because it's derived from 'hysteria', one of the many Greek words for 'womb', only women were thought to experience it.

We think that's a bit of a hysterical response from the men! Don't you?

Hysteria was as much a cop-out for lazy physicians as a form of misogynistic social control. It was diagnosed when a woman exhibited a wide array of symptoms, including anxiety, shortness of breath, fainting, nervousness, sexual desire, insomnia, fluid retention, heaviness in the abdomen, irritability, loss of appetite for food or waining libido, but also, paradoxically, sexually forward behaviour and – our favourite – a tendency to cause trouble for others.

Acute hysteria was blamed when women had sex outside marriage (including masturbation), displayed an attraction to the same sex, or, basically, violated any of the myriad of patriarchal social morals of the time.

Soranus of Ephesus (AD 98–138), the so-called 'father of scientific gynaecology and obstetrics', laid the blame for hysteria on the physical strain of childbirth and recommended women maintain sexual abstinence and perpetual 'virginity' (see page 41). He also suggested that hysterical women should be treated with the utmost care, including with warm baths, and, perhaps our favourite, pelvic massage, but that in extreme cases, the hysterical woman should be forced to enter an insane asylum or undergo a surgical hysterectomy.

FGM

Perhaps the vilest historical and devastating ongoing practice to control women and our sexuality is female genital mutilation (FGM). Although FGM existed long before the nineteenth century, it was rife during this period as a treatment for the symptoms of female hysteria. Removal or cauterization of the clitoris was often prescribed by Western doctors as a cure for everything from masturbation to immorality.

During the late nineteenth century, **JOHN HARVEY KELLOGG** (yes, that is correct, the man who invented the cornflakes you grew up on. That one) was a puritan doctor who actively promoted and performed both a male and female version of circumcision. Not only were cornflakes created as part of a health drive to keep masturbation at bay, he would also recommend applying carbolic acid to the clitoris to reduce any 'abnormal' excitement.

That'll be toast for breakfast, then!

More on FGM throughout history and today on page 121.

MYTH

Rumour has it that, in order to treat the aforementioned female hysteria, doctors would masturbate women to calm their nerves. Complaining of wrist pain, they created the dildo.

TRUTH

While we quite like this idea, the fact is that homemade 'olisbokollikes' – that's dildos to us – have been discovered dating as far back as 30,000 years ago. During a recent prehistoric cave excavation in Germany, scientists discovered what is believed to be the world's oldest dildo – a siltstone phallus with a rounded, polished end and carved rings.

Allegedly, even those pesky ancient Greeks knew the value of dildos for sexual pleasure, making them out of bread in the shape of a baguette, thereby bringing a whole new meaning to the definition of 'yeast infection'.

Although they may not have been called 'dildos' back then, the term 'dildo' was actually first coined in around 1400; originating from the Latin 'dilatare', which means 'open wide', and the Italian for 'delight', which translates as 'diletto' (see vibrators on page 90).

YOU ARE NOT HYSTERICAL: YOU HAVE BEEN IGNORED

While hysteria is no longer a legitimate medical diagnosis (see page 17), these early theories about women's health deeply influenced the development of Western medical science, laying the foundations on which centuries of medical sexism were built and culminating in what is now known as the gender health gap (see page 29). This refers to all the ways in which your gender identity has a bearing on the quality of medical attention you receive and subsequent treatment you might be offered.

The fact that the gender health gap exists is really not that surprising, considering that for centuries in Western societies, doctors were exclusively male and women's bodies were entirely excluded from scientific study. All of this means that we've ended up with a patriarchal healthcare system, one by men, for men, which has treated women's health as secondary and contrived a vast amount of false information about women's bodies. Even as medicine has become more open-minded, the rhetoric still continues. Women's ailments are frequently considered to be psychosomatic and doctors often suggest lifestyle changes rather than exploring adequate diagnostics. Sound familiar? We thought so.

There is another name for this – it's called medical gaslighting. Medical gaslighting is when doctors or medical practitioners blame a patient's illness or symptoms on psychological factors, or even deny the illness entirely. Recent research has found that the combination of a woman's higher pain threshold (yes, this is a scientific fact! – see page 110) and the false assumption that women are emotionally unstable, has left women acutely vulnerable to gaslighting, with repeated misdiagnoses and our pain frequently reported as 'delusional'. Sound a bit like hysteria? It does to us. And just to add insult to injury, when women do receive a decent diagnosis and are prescribed medication, it will likely be medication that has only been tested on male bodies. In a nutshell, women's health concerns have been persistently and consistently invalidated.

IMAGINE A WORLD WHERE GIRLS AND WOMEN ARE TOLD STORIES FOSTERING A SENSE OF PRIDE AND POTENCY IN WHAT IT MEANS TO HAVE A VAGINA. STORIES VALUING FEMALE GENITALIA; STORIES REVEALING THE VAGINA TO BE THE ULTIMATE SYMBOL OF FEMALE POWER. THESE STORIES EXIST: EVERYONE WITH A VAGINA SHOULD KNOW THEM.

RAISING THE SKIRT: THE UNSUNG POWER OF THE VAGINA
DR CATHERINE BLACKLEDGE

THE DISRUPTORS

Early medics may have tried to shroud the vagina by eliminating it from drawings and obscuring it with lies, but throughout history there have been women who have rebelled. They are the disobedient ones, the earth mothers and the wise women who have always been willing to be accused of being irrational, irresponsible and wild. You just need to delve deeper, outside the traditional medical texts we take as gospel, to discover multiple stories of vagina power – from the skirt raisers, witches and healers, and midwives and first female doctors, whose spirit, knowing their rightful place in society, would not be held down.

THE VENUS OF HOHLE FELS

Almost every ancient culture has examples of maternal deities which honour the cycle of life – sexual union, birth, nurture and female creativity.

A recently discovered tiny, ivory statue – The Venus of Hohle Fels (which by the way is thought to be the oldest known representation of the human form) is an extraordinary depiction of a powerful goddess with amplified breasts and vulva, symbolizing the sacred importance of sex and reproduction.

Archaeologists believe that the Hohle Fels Venus is evidence that these societies had a matriarchal social system, where fertility was recognized as the most important aspect of a successful community

SKIRT RAISING

Skirt raising? Yep!

Because at points throughout history, the vulva and vagina have been held in the very highest of esteem. Even in Ancient Greece, before the patriarchy started to evolve, enemies and natural threats like storms were believed to be frightened off by the feminine action of *anasyrma* – or skirt raising.

In the Mediterranean from the twelfth century on, female figures performing *anasyrma* are depicted on armour and stone, baring their powerful sexual organs to keep attackers at bay. This warrior stance was mirrored in the carvings of the sheela na gigs – glorious figures of women; squat, naked, often roaring with laughter and all while pulling open their magnified vulvas – on medieval castles, gateposts and even churches, in Ireland, Britain, France and Spain.

Early historians firmly believed they were a warning against the sins of lust or a talisman against evil. But recently, modern historians in this field have been landing on a far more empowering explanation – that the sheela na gigs actually represented a pre-Christian folk goddess, and the exaggerated labia was an ode to woman's life-giving power and fertility.

We think we might roll with that explanation, don't you?

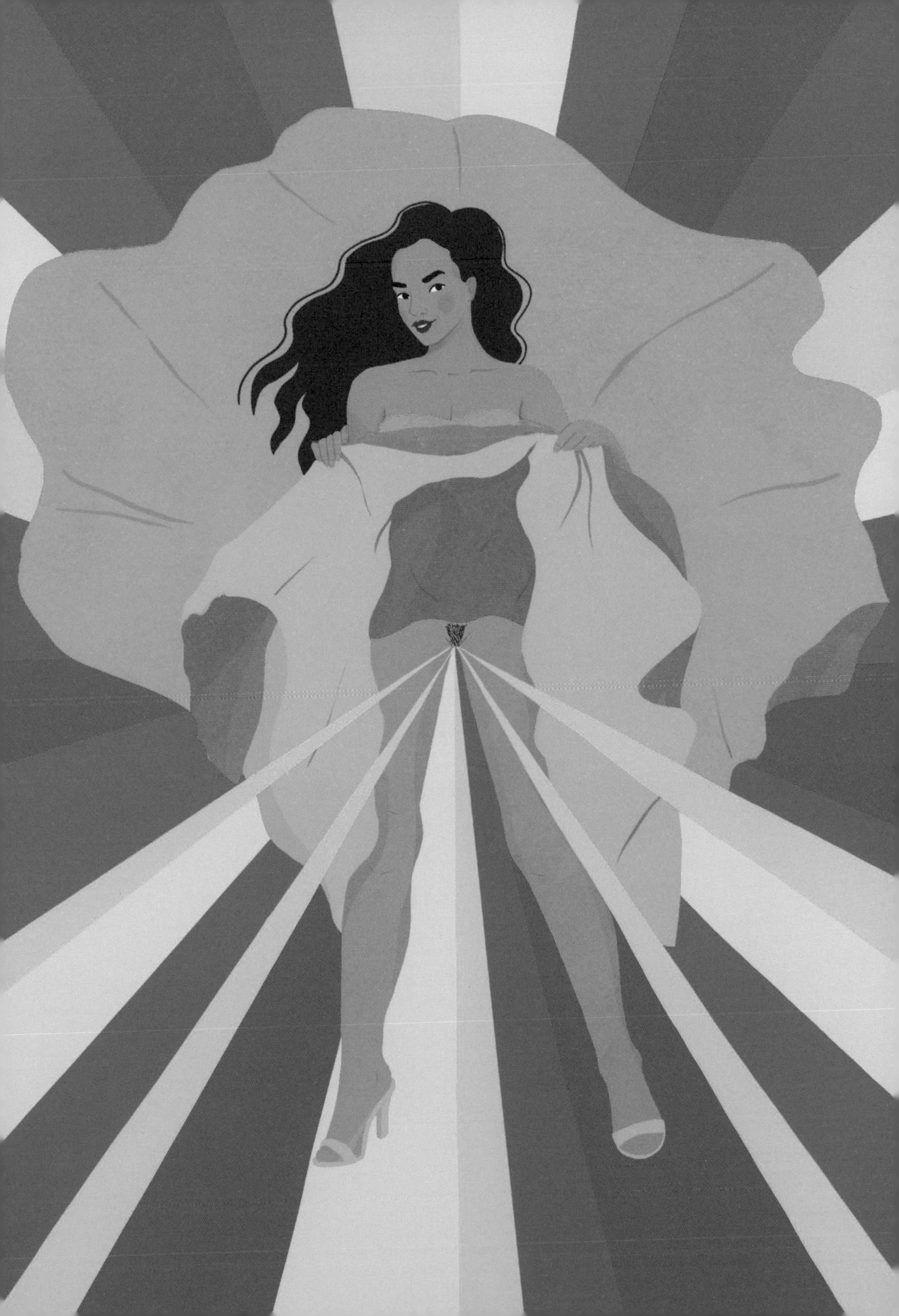

KAPO

Speaking of goddesses, over in Hawaii, Kapo is perhaps the ultimate example of skirt raising.

According to legend, Kapo was a Hawaiian goddess, whose superpower was her flying vagina. The story goes that, one day, Kapo's sister was being assaulted by Kamapua'a, a half-man, half-hog fertility god. Kapo rushed to the rescue the only way she knew how – she lifted her hula skirt with one hand and grabbed her crotch with the other, detaching her vagina. The legend then has it that Kapo's winged vagina flew past Kamapua'a, who was so excited that he started chasing after it. He followed it all the way to the edge of the country, where it landed and left a crater, which Hawaiians named Kohelepelepe ('fringed vulva'), believing it to be the imprint of Kapo's flying vagina.

WITCHES & HEALERS

'WE ARE THE GRANDDAUGHTERS OF THE WITCHES YOU WEREN'T ABLE TO BURN.'
Tish Thawer, *The Witches of BlackBrook*

Next time someone calls you a 'witch' as an insult – thank them for the compliment.

Why? Because for thousands of years, for as long as humans have worshipped deities, witches were honoured as the healers, the wise ones, the seers.

So, when did the term for these ancient female healers become derogatory? In the fifteenth century, during the rise of patriarchal Christianity and capitalism, of course! These new systems could only maintain their male-centric power by demonizing powerful women and witches began to be accused of moral corruption. This included women who were widowed, old, non-churchgoers, landowners, healers and midwives. Many of them were also single and so underpinning much of the rhetoric was a direct attack on female sexuality.

The consequences for being accused of witchcraft were grave – most trials were rigged and often led to death by burning, stoning or hanging. In Europe, between 1500 and 1660, local governments accused and murdered up to 80,000 women for 'witchery' and cast out many more to the lower rungs of society, thereby limiting their economic opportunities and ability to contribute to society.

Then, in the twentieth century, feminists began to reclaim the image of the witch as a symbol of warrior power and the divine feminine. They even campaigned for posthumous pardons for those murdered for being witches. There have been multiple efforts to pardon those wrongfully convicted of witchcraft in the Salem hysteria, with varying degrees of success internationally. Most recently, in 2021, a group of thirteen year olds from North Andover, Massachusetts, won a posthumous pardon for a young woman, Elizabeth Johnson Jr, who was sentenced to death aged twenty two for witchcraft in 1693 during the height of the Salem witchcraft hysteria.

Today, the symbol of the witch is having a renaissance, both spiritually and symbolically, as activists use it to separate themselves from corporate feminism, invoking the witch as a statement of strength and empowerment.

PUSSY

The word 'pussy' has been used to describe the amazing, womanly organ and pleasure centre, otherwise known as the 'vulva', since at least the seventeenth century. From 'petting your pussy' because it likes to be stroked, touched, licked and massaged. With consent. Obvs.

Oh and, FYI – 'pussy' when used in the context of cowardice, is short for 'pusillanimous' not VAGINA!

Pusillanimous: showing a lack of courage or determination; timid.

MIDWIVES

From the beginning of modern medicine, midwives have repeatedly risked their own lives in the fight for women's health.

One of the most legendary is the Athenian Agnodice, who is credited as the first female midwife. Because women at the time were forbidden from practising medicine, Agnodice was forced to disguise herself as a man to work as a physician. As her popularity with female patients grew, rivals accused her of seducing the women of Athens.

Legend has it that, at her trial, she used the *anasyrma* gesture by lifting up her tunic to reveal her identity and save her own life. After testimonials from the women of Athens praised her effective support during childbirth, she was acquitted

Today, women still fight to own our own bodies in childbirth. Ina May Gaskin, one of the leading figures in this field, demands that childbirth be put firmly back in the hands of women and away from what she describes as male-centered, misogynistic birthing processes that still view women's bodies as defective designs and make profit out of women's fears of childbirth and their own bodies.

THAT'S DOCTOR TO YOU!

We may still be a long a way off achieving ultimate health equality in the West (see gender health gap on page 19 and 29), but things started to change, finally, during the Enlightenment (1685–1815) thanks to the invention of the printing press. Printing gave women autonomy, making it possible for us to create our own health guidance, sexual advice literature and midwifery manuals. Even erotica became publicly available for an unprecedented number of female readers. The female health revolution was beginning...

While women had served as physicians and spiritual healers since ancient times, in the West, up until the mid-nineteenth century, there was not one single qualified female doctor.

WHY?

Because women were not allowed to go to medical school, of course!

That all changed in January 1849, when Elizabeth Blackwell, an ambitious, English-born former schoolteacher, graduated from New York's Geneva Medical College and ranked first in her graduating year. **Whoop!**

Blackwell's pioneering spirit extended to her practice. She founded a small clinic in 1853. Many assumed she was simply an abortionist but she battled prejudice against female physicians and the clinic grew into the New York Infirmary for Women and Children in 1857. And in 1868, Blackwell achieved a longheld dream when she opened the Women's Medical College at the infirmary to train more female doctors.

In 1860, Rebecca Davis Lee Crumpler became the first black woman to earn a place at the New England Female Medical College, at a time when most medical schools barred black students, regardless of gender. The school was initially created to train women to work only as midwives, due to the fact that its founder, Samuel Gregory, believed that it was improper for male doctors to assist with childbirth. At the time, many men argued that women were too delicate or not intelligent enough to be doctors. **FFS.** On March 1, 1864, aged 33, Crumpler received a Doctress of Medicine from the New England Female Medical College.

Back across the pond, inspired by meetings with the feminists Emily Davies and Elizabeth Blackwell, suffragette Elizabeth Garrett Anderson became the first woman in Britain to qualify as a physician and surgeon. Unheard of in nineteenth- century Britain, her previous attempts to study at a number of medical schools had all been denied, so with great hutzpah, off she went to enroll as a nursing student at Middlesex Hospital and yet attended the classes solely intended for male doctors instead. Sadly, she was quickly barred following complaints from male students.

Determined as ever, she attended the Society of Apothecaries which did not specifically forbid women from taking their examinations. In 1865, she passed their exams and gained a certificate which enabled her to become a doctor. Soon after, the society changed its rules to prevent other women entering the profession this way. However, still set on obtaining a medical degree and discovering that the University of Paris was allowing women to register, Elizabeth Garrett Anderson promptly taught herself French and headed to France where she successfully earned her degree.

In 1872, Anderson founded the New Hospital for Women in London, staffed entirely by women and appointed her mentor, Elizabeth Blackwell, as the Professor of Gynaecology. Anderson's determination paved the way for other women, and in 1876 an act was passed permitting women to enter the medical profession.

OUR BODIES, OUR SELVES

By the early twentieth century, there was a more established path into medicine for women. Then, during the 1960s and 70s, a new, bolder, movement emerged – the second wave of feminism – and one of its primary aims was to improve healthcare for all women, everywhere.

A significant moment of change was the publication in the US of the pamphlet *Our Bodies, Ourselves*, in 1971. Frustrated by the lack of information for women, twelve feminists from the Boston Women's Collective (now the non profit Our Bodies, Our Selves) collected data, information and filled the 35-cent pamphlet with information on abortion, pregnancy and post-partum depression, revolutionizing women's views on their bodies and sexuality. At a time when the overwhelming majority of gynaecologists were men, *Our Bodies, Ourselves* gave women knowledge and autonomy over their own health, their own bodies. It sold 250,000 copies in New England, USA, alone, with absolutely no marketing. Since its humble beginnings, *Our Bodies, Ourselves* has been published around the globe, translated into 31 languages and the charity in its name continues to develop and promote evidence-based information on girls' and women's reproductive health and sexuality.

THE GENDER HEALTH GAP

Finally, in the 1990s women were included in clinical trials. **WHOOP!**

Yes, exactly, but male bodies are STILL the default in clinical trials today. **YAWN.** Even the standard laboratory mice are male. In 2021, The Medical Research Council, which funds and helps coordinate medical research in Britain, has still failed to produce any guidelines on redefining trials relating to the sex or gender of participants. Thus, for women, access to proper medical care is still, to a certain extent, a gamble.

Today, if you live in a developed country, you are likely to be benefiting from the progress scientists have made since Ancient Greek times in understanding the female body. However, even though the days when a womb was believed to get antsy and wander around the body at will, causing all sorts of trouble are long gone, women's gynaecological health and reproductive systems are still vitally under-researched. This is what has come to be described as the gender health gap, with significant recent research revealing that women's health issues continue to fall victim to the unconscious bias that develops when medical training and testing is still predominantly based on the male form. And we are here to tell you that this is both a national and an international issue. Because even though your healthcare is local to where you live, medical research is conducted globally.

CHAPTER 2

YOUR BODY, YOUR RESPONSIBILITY

ANATOMICAL FACTS AND INSPIRATION

BE YOUR OWN EXPERT

As we've thoroughly outlined in chapter 1, until very recently most aspects of women's healthcare were based on a fierce lack of scientific testing and wild suppositions from the godfathers of the medical patriarchy.

However, through the great perseverance of our prede-sisters (like a predecessor, only strictly female – you heard it here first!), women began to make strides towards equality and today women in many countries can access healthcare that, just a couple of hundred years ago, they didn't even know they needed. But there is still work to do, so while we all beaver away at closing the gender health gap (see page 19 and 29), the ultimate thing you can do to gain power is get to know your own body!

Before we dive any deeper into the female anatomy, we feel we have a responsibility to pause and alert you to a lesser-known and somewhat bizarre fact, that, for all the reasons previously stated, the majority of your intimate female body parts are named after the men that 'discovered' them. **FFS.** As if Dr Ernst Gräfenberg was the first person to find the G spot. We suspect it was more like Mary from Canterbury!

WHEN WOMEN TAKE
CARE OF THEIR HEALTH
THEY BECOME THEIR
OWN BEST FRIEND.

MAYA ANGELOU

THE VULVA

Late Middle English from the Latin 'womb'.

1. PUBIS Also known as the pubic bone, the pubis is the small but mightily protective bone located in front of the pelvic girdle.

2. MONS PUBIS An area of soft protective tissue, the mons pubis covers the pubic bone.

3. CLITERAL HOOD In female human anatomy, the clitoral hood (also called preputium clitoridis and clitoral prepuce) is a fold of skin that surrounds and protects the glans of the clitoris. It also covers the external shaft of the clitoris

4. CLITORIS The clitoris is a female genital organ. It includes erectile tissue, glands, muscles and ligaments, nerves, and blood vessels. The clitoris is much bigger than what you see here (see page 39 for more detail) and is deeply entwined with all of the pelvic structures around it, including the urethra (the duct for urination), the vagina and the labia. For many it is also a place of great pleasure. It comes from the Greek 'kleitoris', which has been translated as both 'little hill' and 'to rub'.

5. VULVA VESTIBULE The tissues located between the vagina and the vulva, comprising the vaginal introitus, make up the vulva vestibule.

6. LABIA MAJORA The prominent pair of cutaneous skin folds that will form the lateral longitudinal borders of the vulval clefts are the labia majora. The folds cover and protect the labia minora, clitoris, vulva vestibule, vestibular bulbs, Bartholin's glands, Skene's glands, urethra, and the vaginal opening.

7. LABIA MINORA The paired folds of smooth tissue underlying the labia majora are the labia minora. Literally the 'minor lips'. Ranging in unique colours from light pink to brownish black. In a sexually unstimulated condition, these tissues cover the vaginal and urethral openings, but when aroused they become more open.

8. URETHRAL OPENING This is a muscular structure in the urethra that helps hold urine inside the body until it's released. The urethra opens into the vestibule, the area between the labia minora. The urethral opening sits just in front of the vaginal opening.

9. VAGINAL OPENING / INTROITUS The vaginal opening, also called the vaginal vestibule or introitus, is the opening into the vagina. It's located between the urethra and the anus. The opening is where menstrual blood leaves the body. It can also be used to birth a baby and for sexual intercourse.

10. PERINEUM The space between the anus and frenulum labiorum pudendi is the perineum. The perineum region of the body between the pubic symphysis (pubic arch) and the coccyx (tail bone), including the perineal body and surrounding structures.

11. ANUS The opening at the lower end of the intestines is the anus. It's where the end of the intestines connect to the outside of the body.

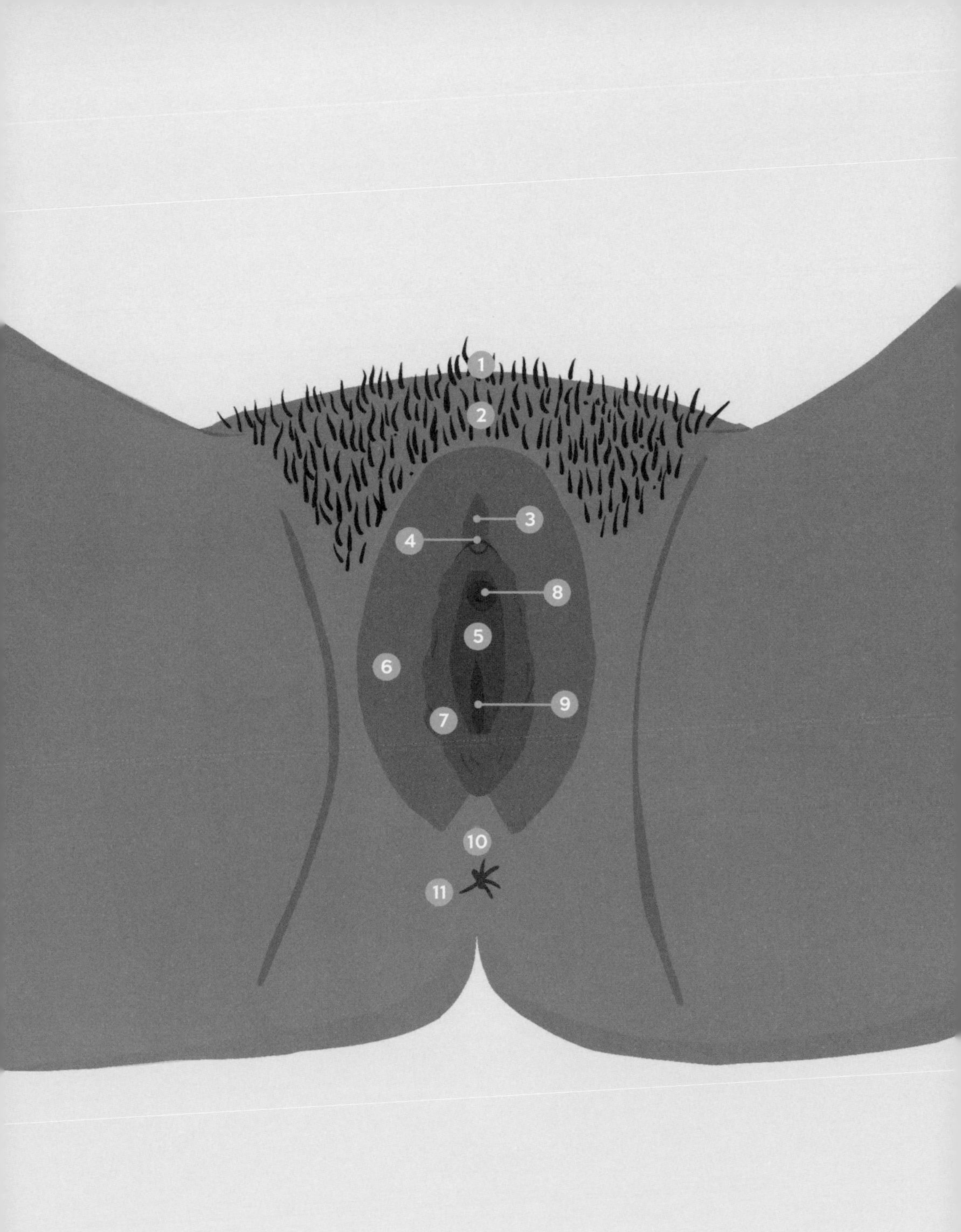
1
2
3
4
8
5
6
9
7
10
11

VIVA LA VULVA

Let's start with the vulva as these are the bits you can see!

The vulva is the external part of the female genitalia and includes the labia, clitoris, vaginal opening and the opening of the urethra. It's there for a reason. Yes, PLEASURE! we hear you roar. It is the place where, for many women, the magic happens, but did you know that the vulva protects the sexual organs, urinary opening, vestibule and vagina as well? In Latin, 'vulva' means 'wrapper'. We are thankful for the wrapper which protects all our sweet spots.

LABIA

In Latin, the word 'labium' means lip. The outer and inner lips of the vulva are, as a pair, called the labia pudenda and then, more specifically, the outer ones are your labia majora and inner ones (sometimes but not always smaller), the labia minora. Just like everything else in your body, the size, shape and colour of labia vary wildly from woman to woman. One side of your labia is almost definitely longer than the other, consistent with the asymmetry of your amazing body, and they will very likely darken with age.

While there is a strong movement towards more realistic representations of all labia, still many women compare theirs to what they see in many anatomical textbooks or pornographic images. Vulvas and labia in traditional porn often look a certain way, but you need to know that many female porn artists have had surgery to create this false so-called 'norm'. Sadly this has left some of us questioning if ours look 'normal' or not and cosmetic surgery to the vulva has been on the rise in recent times. While it is your body and your rules, we hope you know there is no 'normal' standard for how it should look, and we feel passionately about celebrating diverse and beautiful vulvas everywhere!

MYTH

Vulvas all look the same.

BUSTED

In fact, it's the polar opposite! Vulvas are actually like snowflakes – no two are exactly the same. We encourage you to shout this unique fact from the rooftops.

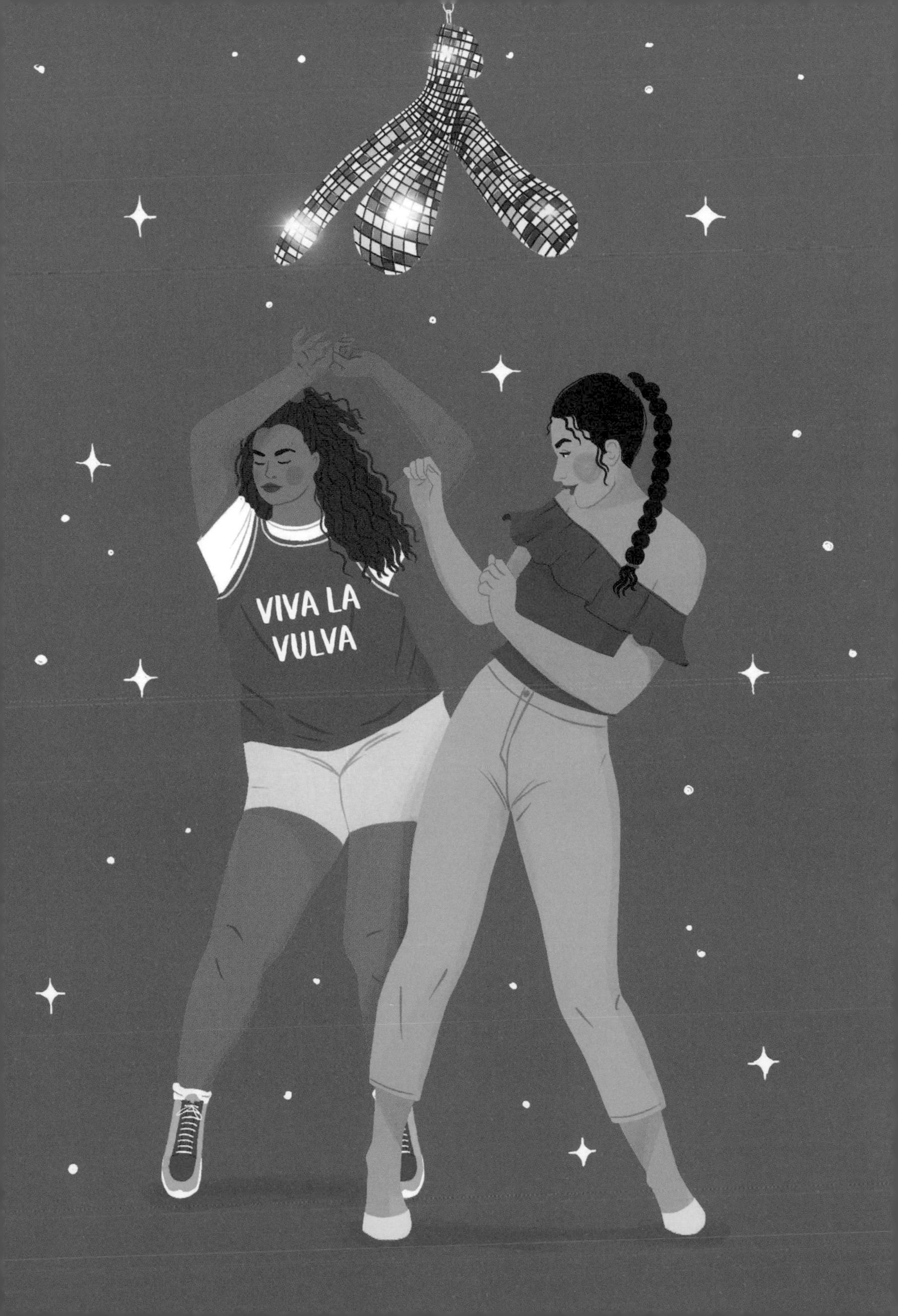
VIVA LA
VULVA

CLITORIS

FYI, the clitoris is an iceberg. An iceberg? Yup!

While it may look small, the part of the clitoris we can see on the vulva is just the tip of this iceberg and the rest of the organ spreads internally and can be as long as 13cm (5in). Found at the top of the vulva, the clitoris is located at the point where the inner labia meet – known as the clitoral hood. The hood is a small flap of mucous tissue that covers and protects the clitoris.

If this amazing anatomy isn't enough to get you excited – here are some other reasons we should all be bowing down to the clitoris.

THE PLEASURE ZONE

That's right, your clitoris is dedicated solely to pleasure. What's more, the clitoris is totally unique as it is the only human organ that's sole function is pleasure. How awesome is that?

ALL-POWERFUL

The glans of the clitoris, we are excited to inform you, has thousands of nerve endings. It's been said, more than double the number of a penis. Not that it's a competition or anything! And just like the penis, the clitoris becomes erect, due to increased blood flow, when aroused.

INFINITE

Did you know that your clitoris actually grows as you get older? After menopause, the clitoris can become two and a half times larger than it was during your teenage years, and seven times larger than it was at birth.

TIMELESS

No matter how much wear and tear your clitoris may experience over the years, it doesn't age, which means it retains all of its pleasure capacity.

GROUNDBREAKING

The least interesting thing that makes it unique? The word 'clitoris' is actually borrowed directly from Greek when we usually rely on Latin for our formal words relating to sex.

CLITORAL ABUSE

Despite these phenomenal facts placing the clitoris right at the top of the anatomical hierarchy, devastatingly it has been continuously and repeatedly demonized in many cultures. We've already mentioned those pesky Ancient Greeks, who thought that it was an abnormality (see page 12). But you should also know that Sigmund Freud, the father of psychoanalysis who had a huge influence on 20th-century thinking about sex, famously considered clitoral orgasms to be 'immature' compared to vaginal orgasms. Yep, we'll just let that sink in for a minute when we know that the majority of women who can climax, climax through clitoral stimulation.

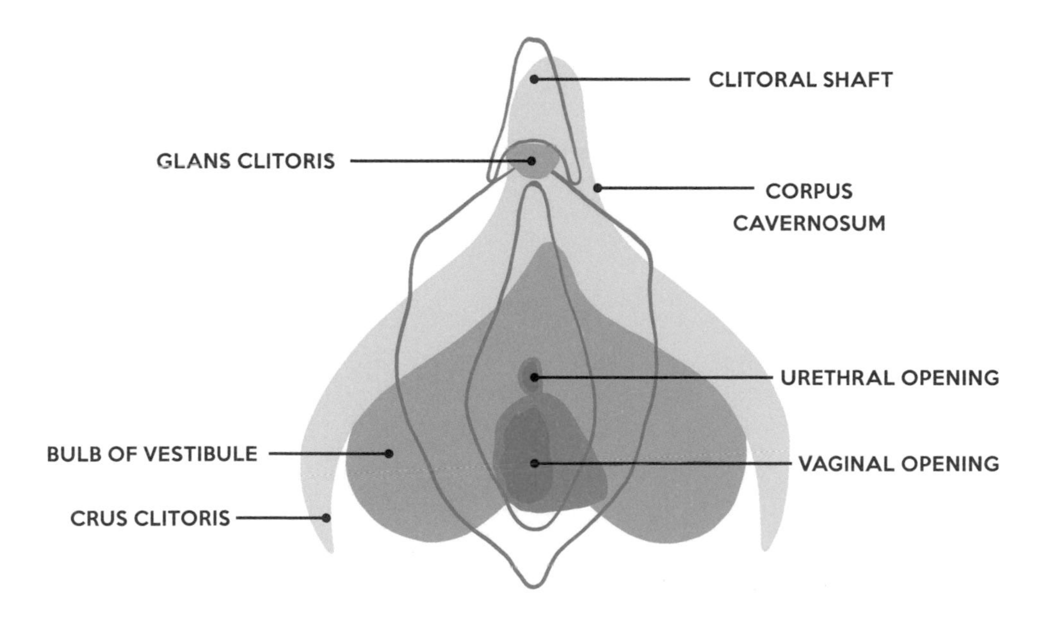

Perhaps the greatest revelation of our generation is the full breadth of the previously ignored clitoris. We must thank the scientists who have spent hours searching for the supposed mythical, highly erogenous G-spot for this. Their research has revealed exciting, new anatomical relationships and dynamic interactions between the clitoris, urethra and anterior vaginal wall leading to an entirely new concept – the ClitoUrethroVaginal (CUV) complex. The what? In layman's terms this is a variable, multifaceted area that, when stimulated during penetration, could induce orgasmic responses. OMG YES!

What's perhaps even more exciting is that this enhanced knowledge of the anatomy and physiology of the CUV complex should help to avoid the centuries of damage that has been done to women's bodies during surgical procedures.

VAGINA

Let's get our facts straight shall we? The vagina comprises the internal female genitals. It is the muscular tube that runs from the vulva, all the way up to the cervix. Every vagina is unique but, providing there are no medical problems, it is through this tube that menstrual blood and, if you choose, babies leave our bodies.

As might be expected, the word 'vagina' is Latin. In Latin, it originally meant 'sheath' or 'scabbard', presumably for a sword to sit in. This symbolizing of the vagina as being a mere vessel for the penis is one of the greatest misconceptions. EVER. Your vagina is, in fact, a marvel of physiological engineering – profoundly strong yet wildly flexible, to enable the most important role of the human anatomy – **the survival of the species.**

HYMEN HYPE

We hate to break it to you, but your hymen has been given way too much kudos.

Long heralded as an indicator of 'virginity', the hymen is simply small folds of mucous tissue that sit 1–2cm (0.3–0.7in) inside the vaginal opening. It is, of course, uniquely shaped in every female. Many women are in fact born with very little hymenal tissue, so it seems like they don't have a hymen at all.

It is true that, for some women, the tissue can break or tear upon first sexual intercourse (or other penetration), or it could stretch; but it absolutely doesn't always as a matter of course. All of this means, of course, that the presence or absence of a hymen says nothing about whether a woman has had sex or not.

The hymen was named after the Greek god of marriage and so recently a group of vulva warriors in Sweden renamed it the 'vaginal corona' in order to reclaim it and, in doing so, dissipate many of the misogynistic myths around female virginity.

POPPING THE CHERRY

The euphemism 'popping the cherry' has been around since the 1970s to describe the moment a woman loses her virginity. It comes from the word 'pop', which was used with a sexual connotation as early as the 1600s and alluded to the breaking of a woman's hymen during sex, which may slightly bleed, evoking the red colour of the cherry. REWIND! There is no cherry, there is no popping. YOU ARE NOT A FRUIT!

THE MYTH OF VIRGINITY

In most cultures, the word 'virgin' refers to somebody who has not had penetrative sex. In some more extreme societies, masturbation is also included. But we have some news for you – **virginity is a social construct.**

Pause for a moment and think about it – it only exists because we've all agreed to it.

This global myth has been created to keep women trapped in a purity shame cycle. It goes like this – women are raised to believe their power lies in their beauty and sexual prowess, and yet this power should be withheld because when it is infiltrated in an untimely way (i.e. before a man chooses her as his lifelong companion), she will be 'soiled'. This dichotomy leads women and girls to experience deep-rooted confusion about how we should take up space on the planet and, perhaps worse, provides a fertile ground for slut-shaming when a woman doesn't adhere to society's absurd demands on her frigidity.

But guess what – we can stop this right now.

Stop saying 'I lost my virginity to...' and start saying 'the first person I had sex with was...'

Because when you have sex for the first time, you do not actually lose anything. Most likely, it will have been a deeply important moment for you in your personal development as a human. Furthermore, it is impossible to lose something that is just a made-up construct. In a nutshell, having sex for the first time should not affect in any way your 'worth'.

Also, for the record, young men have an equally challenging time but in the other direction. They often have to deal with the immense pressure that they should be sexually active in order to prove themselves.

THE CERVIX

Small but oh-so-powerful, the cervix is a tube-shaped passage at the bottom of the uterus that connects to the vagina. It's about 5cm (2in) long and, although it's very narrow, it is able to dilate vastly during labour.

Prior to childbirth, it is your cervix that produces the clear, slippery mucus during ovulation that helps sperm swim from the vagina into the uterus so that the egg can choose one to fertilize with. Yes that is correct – the egg chooses the sperm (more on that later; see page 71).

Then, if conception happens, that mucus thickens and plugs up the cervix, preventing microbes and other potentially harmful agents from hurting the developing foetus. Finally, when it's time to give birth, the cervical plug discharges again, and the cervix itself dilates to approximately 10cm (4in) so that a small human can make it safely into the world. After stretching, the cervix will usually return to its original size. This can take up to six weeks in some cases.

MYTH

If a woman has too much sex, her vagina becomes 'loose'.

TRUTH

Utter biological nonsense. This is commonly known as slut-shaming and it needs to stop! The vagina is actually deeply clever and can stretch in size for different reasons, such as sex and childbirth, but it doesn't stay that way. After the fact, it returns to its normal size, kind of like an elastic band, and the walls, when dormant, often rest against each other.

SQUALENE

Natural vaginal lubricant is composed of sweat, sebum, cervical mucus, exfoliated cells, urea, acetic and lactic acids, complex alcohols, ketones and squalene.

Squalene can also be found in sharks. Sharks? Exactly! Both vaginas and sharks contain squalene, which should come as no surprise to anyone who knows the true power of the **VAGINA!**

A naturally-occurring substance found in plants, animals and humans, squalene, is synthesized in the liver, then circulated in the bloodstream to keep our skin hydrated and assist with vaginal lubrication. For a long time, it was also commercially extracted from shark livers and was the number one ingredient in many anti-ageing moisturizers (until a clever scientist created a man-made version and saved the sharks!).

The planet's natural moisturizer is not only found in sharks and humans – it is also present in olives, rice bran and sugarcane.

Need a moment to change that supermarket order?

YONI

'Yoni' is a Sanskrit word that in literal translation means 'womb' or – 'THE SOURCE'. It can also be used to describe the female sexual organs such as vagina and vulva.

DISCHARGE

Hate discharge? We suggest you learn to love it! The fluid released by glands in the vagina and cervix, discharging water, bacteria and vaginal cells is, in fact, your daily self-cleaning mechanism. The fluid carries dead cells and bacteria out of the body, and vaginal discharge helps keep the vagina clean and prevent infection. Thank the discharge!

pH

The pH of a substance is a measurement of how acidic or basic it is, on a scale of 0 to 14, with the lower numbers representing greater acidity. Vaginal pH is a measure of the acidity of the vaginal environment and in healthy women vaginal pH is typically 3.5 to 4.5. This is quite acidic – about as acidic as beer or tomatoes – and busy microbe communities in the vagina maintain this acidity.

Studies show that vaginal issues often occur when vaginal pH is unbalanced. This means that microorganisms can flourish, causing vaginal odor and sometimes discomfort. An elevated pH can be caused by normal everyday events. Period blood, for example, has a pH of 7.4, and hormone fluctuations caused by the menopause and pregnancy also have an impact.

IT'S ALL ABOUT BALANCE

See the list below for top tips on how to keep your pH level balanced.

SEX If your are enjoying heterosexual, penetrative, condom-free sex and you notice a change in your discharge, try douching with water afterwards! Semen has a pH of 7.1 to 8.

DO NOT USE HYGIENE PRODUCTS! Even soap can have a pH of over 8.

TAMPONS, because they retain the blood fluids, can cause pH to rise. Do not leave them in too long!

DIET – nope, not the 'I need to be thinner' kind. We don't believe in those at The Happy Vagina – but the eat for your vagina kind. Fill your vagina with plenty of fruits, vegetables and wholegrains (not literally of course!).

DRINK WATER! Not only does this help to regulate the body's natural cleansing systems, it's also quite handy when it comes to sex (more on that later; see page 97).

VAGINAL STEAMING

Vaginal steaming is an ancient ritual that regained fame in 2017. However, on deeper investigation, it turns out your vulva doesn't really need steaming, after all. Specialized vagina spa treatments may seem intriguing but unless part of a Goddess self-care ritual, they're, at best, unnecessary and, at worst, could lead to infections or even burns on your most sensitive parts.

While your preferences are between you and YOU, we say save your spa budget for a facial-facial instead.

THE OVARIES

A strong contender for the most amazing organ in a woman's body, the ovaries have two main responsibilities. Firstly, providing there are no medical difficulties, every 28 days they produce the eggs, or ovum, from which all of life stems. When you put it like that – **WOW!** Yes, we know!

A beautiful greyish-pink in colour, they have an uneven surface caused by cystic structures, which are completely normal due to the different stages of egg growth and development. The size of the ovaries changes depending on a woman's age; larger during her reproductive phase and shrinking after menopause.

The ovaries are also one of the major areas of the body where hormones are produced and secreted; oestrogen and progesterone, to be exact, which stimulate the female reproductive organs and initiate puberty and the menopause.

Amazing, right? This is how it works:

During the first part of your menstrual cycle, before ovulation, the ovaries produce mainly oestrogen. Oestrogen is responsible for the development of female reproductive organs and the menstrual cycle. After ovulation, production focuses mainly on progesterone, which helps maintain a normal menstrual cycle.

OVARIAN POPS

Often referred to as *mittelschmerz* – that's mid-cycle pain to you and me! – ovarian pain that's associated with ovulation is often caused by the growth of the follicle (which holds the maturing egg) stretching the surface of the ovary. If you're tuned into your body, you might feel this as a twinge or pop.

EGGS 'N' OVULATION

Even though women have been menstruating since before homo sapiens were fully evolved as a species, it wasn't until the nineteenth century that scientists linked periods to ovulation.

The nineteenth century?! **FFS.** Yes, we know!

Women actually begin life with 6–7 million eggs – even when we are still a micro-sized foetus in the womb. And because you have two ovaries, ovulation can but does not necessarily always alternate back and forth between them each cycle.

WOMB

Also known as the uterus, the facts are these:

The womb is a hollow, pear-sized muscular organ in a woman's lower abdomen, perched between the bladder and the rectum. The narrow, lower portion of the uterus is the cervix or the neck of your uterus. The broader upper part is called the the 'corpus', which means 'entirety' or 'whole'.

The womb really is one of the most incredible organs in a human being: the strongest muscle in the body by weight and filled with unlimited sexual and creative power. During pregnancy, a woman's uterus expands from being tucked behind the pubic bone, to being as large as a helium balloon, reaching all the way to the ribcage and stretching the abdomen outwards visibly. Then, when it's done, it shrinks back down. **WILD!**

The womb is also the only organ that can grow another organ within it – the placenta, the life-giving channel which feeds the foetus through pregnancy via its attachment to the uterine wall of the mother and to the baby through the umbilical cord.

MYTH

A baby is born with all the eggs she will ever have.

TRUTH

This commonly-held scientific dogma regarding the female biological clock – that women are born with all their eggs and that these eggs slowly expire as we move from birth to menopause – is utter nonsense. Over the past decade, a series of revolutionary experiments have suggested that oocyte cells (that's an immature ovum, or egg cell to us) can in fact regenerate after birth.

THE BUSH

That'll be female pubic hair, when left in its natural state.

Up until the middle of the last century, The Bush was still a literary euphemism, echoing other countryside metaphors, like undergrowth, ling, thicket, garden and flower, all of which have been used in the same way for many centuries. The Romans referred to female pubic hair as a fern and the Greeks as a rose bush.

Today, The Bush has become an everyday colloquialism, gaining considerable traction in mainstream press and regaining popularity with women worldwide.

Did you know that your pubic hair tends to fall out after about three weeks? That's just a fraction of the life expectancy of the hair on your head, which can hang around for up to seven years.

> **'YOU'RE SUPPOSED TO TREAT IT LIKE THE BEAUTIFUL FLOWER IT IS. WATERING IT. FERTILIZING IT. IT NEEDS NOURISHMENT. IT'S HUNGRY.'**
> Cameron Diaz

We couldn't agree more Ms Diaz.

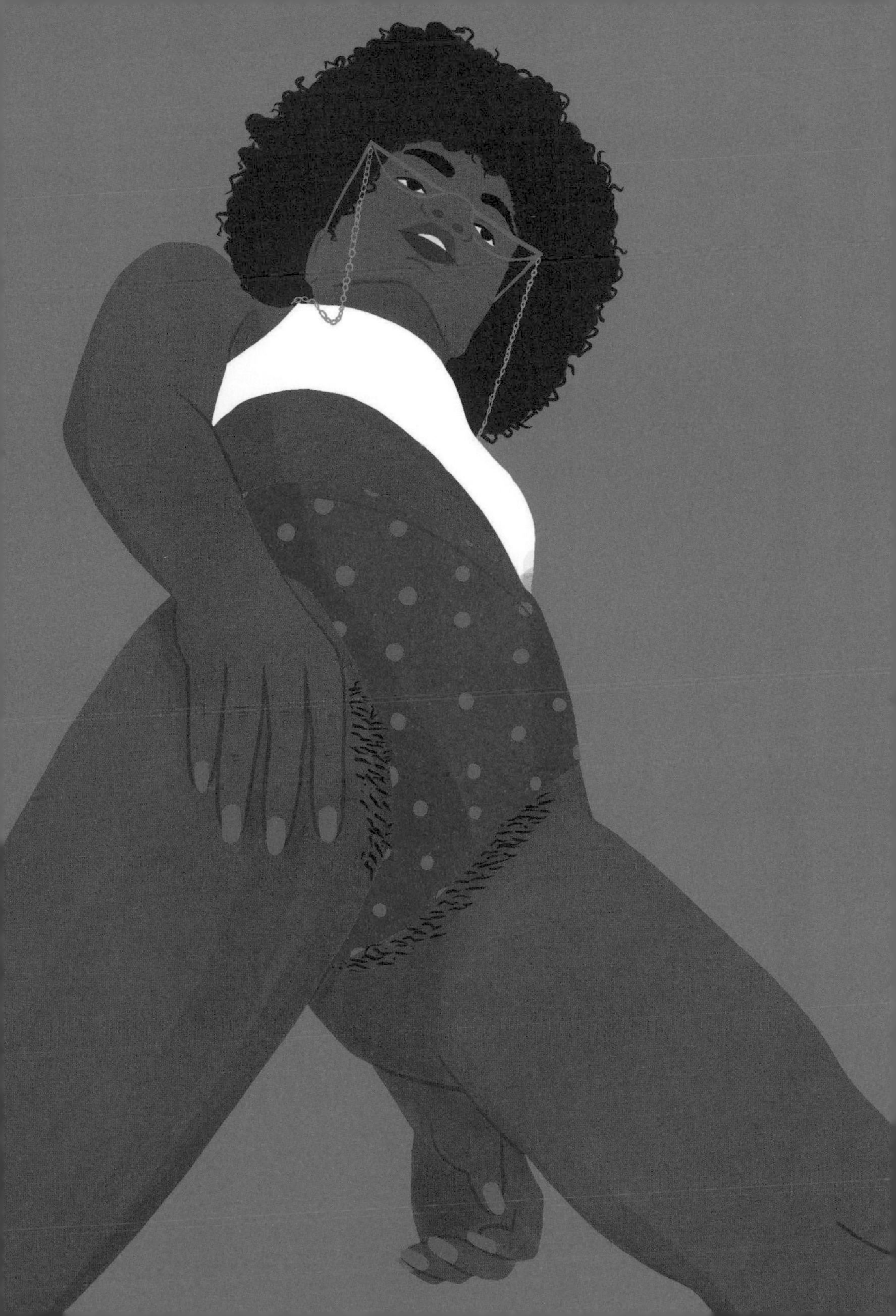

THE HISTORY OF HAIR REMOVAL

Hair removal for aesthetic reasons has been around for centuries. Back in ancient Egypt, women considered all body hair uncivilized and used a homemade sugar wax to remove their pubic hair, while over in Rome in the sixth century BC, upper-class women used tweezers and pumice stones. In England, Elizabethan women removed their eyebrows and hair from their foreheads to give themselves a longer brow. Then, over the centuries, as clothing fashions changed and arms and legs became more exposed, hair removal gained further popularity. The shortage of nylon stockings during World War II consolidated the trend as more women began to shave their legs.

With the introduction of the bikini in 1946, women began to trim their pubic hair again. Feminists of the 1960s and 1970s rebelled and brought back the bush, but the rebellion was short-lived when, in the 1980s, the Brazilian wax exploded onto the beauty scene.

Shave, don't shave, mix it up, but be aware that a cleanly shaven body is more open to infections (see page 104).

And also bear in mind that fashions are often created to make us buy products. So, most of all, be yourself, everyone else is taken! (See page 106).

MERKIN

What's a merkin? A pubic wig.

These items still exist and today are mostly used in the entertainment industry. In the film *Dr Strangelove*, the name of the president of the USA was chosen with some care; he was called Merkin Muffley.

However, in previous centuries, they were especially popular when the treatment for lice and also venereal diseases, like syphilis, involved shaving off the pubic hair.

Which brings us finally to the...

MUFF

Or perhaps, more accurately, the female genitalia! So, why 'muff'? Well, apparently the word muff originally specifically referred to the pubic hair, but it has been used in this wider sense since at least the seventeenth century. Cunnilingus is sometimes called 'muff-diving'. For more on cunnilingus, see page 91.

KNOWLEDGE IS POWER

While hysteria – which, by the way, was only finally removed from the American Psychiatric Association's list of modern diseases in 1952 – seems relatively archaic today, women are STILL frequently misdiagnosed and mistreated by both male and female physicians (see medical gaslighting on page 19). So, the ultimate power is to become an expert in your own body.

How to develop your inner expert:

ESTABLISH A GOOD RELATIONSHIP WITH YOUR DOCTOR

A great physician will look for health in your body rather than just treating disease. But it is also your responsibility to build this relationship. Stop going to the doctor only when there is something wrong. Instead, book a yearly check up.

PREVENTION IS KEY

Does your family have a history of potentially hereditary conditions? If so, educate yourself on them and let your doctor know so that you can get any regular screening tests you need.

KNOW YOUR NORMAL

Last but definitely not least, make sure you know all your body's glorious rhythms and idiosyncracies. Then, if your symptoms get dismissed, you can be articulate and push back, requesting tests because you know things are out of sorts.

DO NOT FEAR THE SMEAR

We know it can be uncomfortable but we urge you – do not fear the smear – your health is too precious. While so many parts of the female anatomy are still misunderstood, with their related conditions often going undiagnosed for far too long, we just want to take a moment to be grateful for the smear test, also known as the PAP test or cervical screening.

HPV

The human papillomavirus (HPV) is the most common sexually transmitted infection (STI) and it is estimated that almost every sexually active woman will be infected with one or more types of this virus at some point in her life. Most of the time, your body mounts a strong defence against HPV and clears it before it does any harm. However, some types of HPV can alter the cells of your cervix and, over many years, these changes can lead to cervical cancer if not detected and treated. Luckily, we have excellent methods of early detection through smear/PAP tests, which involve your doctor or nurse swabbing your cervix to detect the presence of abnormal cells.

QUIM

Recently rescued back into common usage by feminist pornographic literature, this ancient word - meaning the female genitals - had all but fallen into obscurity earlier in the twentieth century.

It may be related to the Anglo-Saxon 'cweman' and hence to 'cwithe' meaning 'womb', or possibly to the Celtic 'cwm' - a cleft or valley. Although the first explanation is by far the most likely, the second is supported by the large number of words for a cleft or gash that are used as euphemisms for vagina.

The noun 'quim' was also a Victorian word used to refer to the fluids produced by the vagina, specifically during orgasm.

RED FLAGS TO LOOK OUT FOR:

FREQUENT NEED TO PEE

You might have noticed that you urinate more regularly at specific points in the menstrual cycle, especially just before your period or around ovulation. This is totally normal! Outside of that, the average should be around four and ten times a day. More than that could be a sign of diabetes, a urinary tract or bladder condition or, when combined with other symptoms, some cancers. You know the drill… make that appointment and, if you don't feel listened to, demand some tests!

VAGINAL ITCHING

Vaginal itching can be a nuisance, but it is often just caused by hormonal changes and rights itself with no intervention. If it doesn't go away or you have severe symptoms accompanied by abnormal discharge, bleeding or burning with urination, get it checked out!

ABNORMAL VAGINAL DISCHARGE

Vaginal discharge is to be thanked (see page 43). However, there are certain types of discharge that can indicate a yeast or bacterial infection. These sometimes need a bit of nutritional or medical help to clear up but are often easily treatable. If your discharge looks unusual or smells foul, get a proper diagnosis and treatment plan!

VAGINAL BLEEDING

Abnormal vaginal bleeding may be minor, and can be very common post-sex, in between periods or if you use a hormone-based contraceptive, but it could also indicate something more sinister. If it continues, you must make an appointment with your doctor immediately to rule out conditions like cervical cancer or STIs, like chlamydia.

PELVIC PAIN

Do not ignore chronic or repetitive pelvic pain. We know it can be similar to menstrual cramps – and you may even feel your follicles popping at ovulation – but it's imperative you get it checked out and demand tests if its recurring and impacting your quality of life. It could be a symptom of endometriosis (a disease that currently takes up to seven years to diagnose **WTF**) or cancer.

CHAPTER 3

ANYTHING YOU CAN DO, **I CAN DO** BLEEDING

PERIODS AND HORMONES

THE CURSE

Let's get something straight: your menstrual cycle is NOT a curse. It's the biological rhythm that allows us to bring new life into the world. Which is amazing, obviously. So, where did this 'curse' myth come from? One likely source is the Bible's 'Curse of Eve' (Genesis 3:16), during which God, with his characteristic beneficence, says to Eve:

'I will greatly multiply thy sorrow and thy conception: in sorrow thou shalt bring forth children; and thy desire shall be to thy husband, and he shall rule over thee'.

We say, 'Whatever!' and are here to share with you a whole heap of amazing facts about your period and everything it brings with it!

BOW DOWN TO THE PERIOD

Periods are amazing. Period.

Part of the menstrual cycle, periods are the few days mid-cycle when women, and people who menstruate, bleed from the vagina. Most people have menstrual periods that last four to seven days, around every 28 days or so, but can range from day 21 to day 40.

Rich with stem cells and responsible for bringing life into the world, it is now time to smash all stigma and bow down to the period.

Each month during the so-called 'fertile years', a woman's body creates a rich endometrial layer in the womb in preparation to grow and nourish a whole new human being. More commonly than not, a baby is not conceived and a woman's body will return to its regular rhythm. How? By releasing this extremely valuable and nutritive goddess substance during the menstrual cycle. And when we say goddess, we really do mean goddess, because women's menstrual cycles and the stages of our fertile journeys, whatever they look like, reflect the glorious cycles of the Earth, Moon and Sun. Let's go a little deeper...

The moon cycle is 29.5 days and the average woman's menstrual cycle is 29.5 days.

The average age for the menopause to start is 52, which is also the number of weeks in a year.

There are an average of four weeks in a women's menstrual cycle and there are four seasons in a year.

CYCLICAL HISTORY

Back in the 1800s, the average age a young woman would start menstruating was around seventeen. Nowadays, the average age most girls start their period is twelve but that is getting younger in some countries. There are a few key reasons for this, one of which is improved nutrition. We're eating better and more than our ancestors did and fat cells make oestrogen. The more fat cells you have, the more oestrogen you have in your body, which can trigger the start of your menstrual cycle. Increased stress levels are also a factor. That's right, high stress levels can actually trigger the beginning of your period. Finally, the other factor is your father's hormones. Yes, you read that correctly, there is some evidence to show that a father being at home stops his daughter's hormones from maturing.

NOT A DIRTY WORD

VAGINA, VAGINA, VAGINA! It's not a dirty word, and yet the first movie to use the word 'vagina' on film was Disney's *The Story of Menstruation*, released in 1946.

LET'S GET DOWN TO GODDESSES

In your lifetime, providing you don't have any challenges or decide to use hormones to stop your bleeds, you will have somewhere between 400 to 450 periods. Isn't that wild?! Add that up and it's approximately ten years. Yes, you will spend TEN years of your life bleeding. That's 3,500 days menstruating. Want some more wild facts? OK, buckle up...

We know that the clever menstrual cycle is also rather changeable, but did you know that cold weather can make a period heavier and longer than usual? During the winter months, a woman's flow, period duration and even pain level are greater than in the summer. This pattern also extends to women who live in colder rather than warmer climates.

The seasons can also affect your PMT too – the darker, shorter days can adversely impact your mood when combined with female reproductive hormones. This is thought to be because of a lack of sunshine, which helps our bodies to produce vitamin D and dopamine, which boost our moods, happiness, concentration and all-round health levels.

And your menstrual cycle can also have a profound effect on your body. Ever noticed that you get more attention when you're coming into your flow? Well, that's because the reproductive hormones affect your natural scent, meaning you smell different when you're on your period. While this is very subtle, it harks back to our caveman days when men would be more attracted to women who were ovulating rather than menstruating; meaning they could procreate. **Wild, right?!**

And what's more, periods can also change your vocal tone. According to researchers, women's voices can change slightly during their menstrual cycles due to reproductive hormones affecting the vocal cords.

PRAISE THE PERIOD!

In India, there's a yearly festival that celebrates the annual period of the goddess Kamakhya. For four days in June, Shakti pilgrims (a denomination of Hinduism) gather in Assam from miles around to celebrate Ambubachi Mela, a four-day fertility festival.

PERIOD PREJUDICE

OK, so now we know that periods are not just some basic biological process – in fact, without them there is no life! But historically, periods have not always been favoured so well. If you dig deep, the list of endless vile and misogynistic myths that were created about periods by uneducated, fear-filled humans is terrifying. So, we've picked out some of our favourites to save you the trauma!

THE MOST OUTRAGEOUS FALSE PROCLAMATION ABOUT PERIODS. EVER.

As we mentioned, once upon a time it was believed that the period was a curse and, over time, all sorts of fear-based lies have been told about it. Perhaps one of the most ridiculous was in the 1920s when an esteemed doctor – the Hungarian-born American pediatrician, Béla Schick – suggested that flowers would wilt and bread wouldn't rise if held in close proximity to a menstruating human. This was all due to an imaginary poisonous toxin called menotoxin.

HA! We'll just give you a moment to recover, shall we?

While it seems funny now, the devastating reality is that this wasn't just a wacky theory – it was an extremely serious debate. Eventually, of course, it was proved wrong and everyone agreed that menstruating women did not, after all, release an invisible poison.

But here's the rub – this view did persist in science through the twentieth century and sadly, today in many cultures it is still believed that a menstruating person is unclean. Women within these communities are asked to isolate, sometimes sent to menstrual huts and often banned from participating in group activities, like cooking, studying and praying. Exiled from the comfort of their homes to barebone huts, these women's lives are put at risk every month from snake bites, physical assaults and freezing temperatures during the winter months. And then there is the ongoing mental health issues women in these cultures continue to experience, as a result of being so deeply shamed about their periods.

See page 120 for international charities campaigning for period equality.

WE NEED TO BOW TO THE PERIOD, WITHOUT IT THERE IS NO HUMANITY.

JUNE SARPONG ON THE HAPPY VAGINA PODCAST

TOADS, TAMPONS & OTHER SANITARY PRODUCTS

So, how should you manage this free-flowing goddess blood?

Today, we are lucky enough to be able to support our menstrual flow with pads, tampons, menstrual cups, reusable period pants or, if we choose, even hormones that shut down the period altogether. But it hasn't always been quite this simple.

Historically, women were forced to be more creative. In medieval Europe, folklore suggested that, if your flow was extremely heavy, the go-to cure was to find a toad, burn it in a pot, and then wear the ashes in a pouch near your vagina. Somebody call animal welfare!

Other, perhaps more rational, forms of historical sanitary products included softened papyrus, lint wrapped around wood, paper, knitted pads, rabbit fur and even grass. But by the late nineteenth century – at around the same time as women in the West were demanding a seat at the medical table – things started to look up and menstrual belts with loops of elastic and thick cotton pads to clip or pin on were made available.

Then, finally, the first decent menstrual care product was created by French nurses on the battlefield during the First World War. Realizing that the disposable cellulose bandages they used on wounded soldiers absorbed blood better than cotton, were inexpensive and easy to dispose of, these women started using them for their period flow. Commercial manufacturers quickly caught on and the first disposable pads were made available for purchase in 1888. But marketing them was as difficult as trying to use the hashtag **#vagina** on Instagram.

Women were still sitting on a vast amount of historical shame about periods and many felt uncomfortable buying a product named 'sanitary ware'. The commercial advertizing landscape, which started in the early 1940s and exploded in the 1950s was no better. An advert that mentioned the word 'vagina' was pulled after three networks refused to show it. They replaced 'vagina' with 'down there' but even that didn't make it past the censors.

The advert, which finally ran as part of a campaign in 2010, was still not allowed to mention the vagina. Even in the twenty-first century, the life-giving parts of our bodies are still being forced into invisibility.

PERIOD POVERTY

Period poverty affects people who menstruate all over the world and not just in poorer countries. Menstrual products are expensive and so anywhere there is poverty, you will find women struggling to support their own bleed. Quite frankly, we believe period care should be free for all women, but it is not just the lack of access to products that creates period poverty.

Research has shown that women and girls will miss school, work and social gatherings when there is not a safe and hygienic space to support them during their bleed. This of course negatively impacts on education, mental health and overall quality of life.

If you are in the privileged position of enjoying the multiple options of period care on the market today from pants to cups, think about supporting a charity that helps those that can't. See page 120 for our suggestions!

THE TAMPON

A plug of cotton inserted into the vagina, named after the verb 'tamp', meaning to stop up a hole, or to ram home the charge in a barrel-loading gun. Lovely!

The first tampons were made with a sewing machine and a compression machine, which compacted the absorbent material.

A woman who uses tampons could use up to 11,000 in her lifetime.

MENSTRUATION
IS LIKE A
SUPERPOWER.

ELIZABETH BANKS

PERIOD STRESS

As we previously mentioned, the majority of our female anatomy has been named after the men who apparently 'discovered' it. But not the commonly used term 'premenstrual syndrome'. This was finally defined in 1953 by the British female physician Dr Katharina Dalton. Hallelujah!

Way back in the first century, the Greek physician Soranus mentioned in his guide for midwives that women possibly became tense before their periods but no-one in the medical field had any idea what caused this tension until, finally, in 1931 it was linked to the ovarian cycles.

1931? **WTF.** We know! But then, when you think the ovarian follicles weren't even located until the mid-seventeenth century by Regnier de Graaf, it's not really that surprising. Graaf's research was also lacking, due to insufficient microscopic equipment, and it was not until 1827 (150 years later!) that Karl Ernst von Baer first identified the ovum.

However, back to you, and the present day – premenstrual tension can be debilitating. Symptoms can include anything from mood swings, anxiety, bloating, pain and skin irritation to reduced or increased appetite – for both food and sex.

There are things you can do to support yourself, like resting and drinking lots of water, taking regular exercise, eating a healthy diet and prioritizing kindness. Yes, that is correct; our top tip for PMT is **be kind to yourself.**

Oh yes and – keep a track of when it's coming. For yourself and everyone around you!

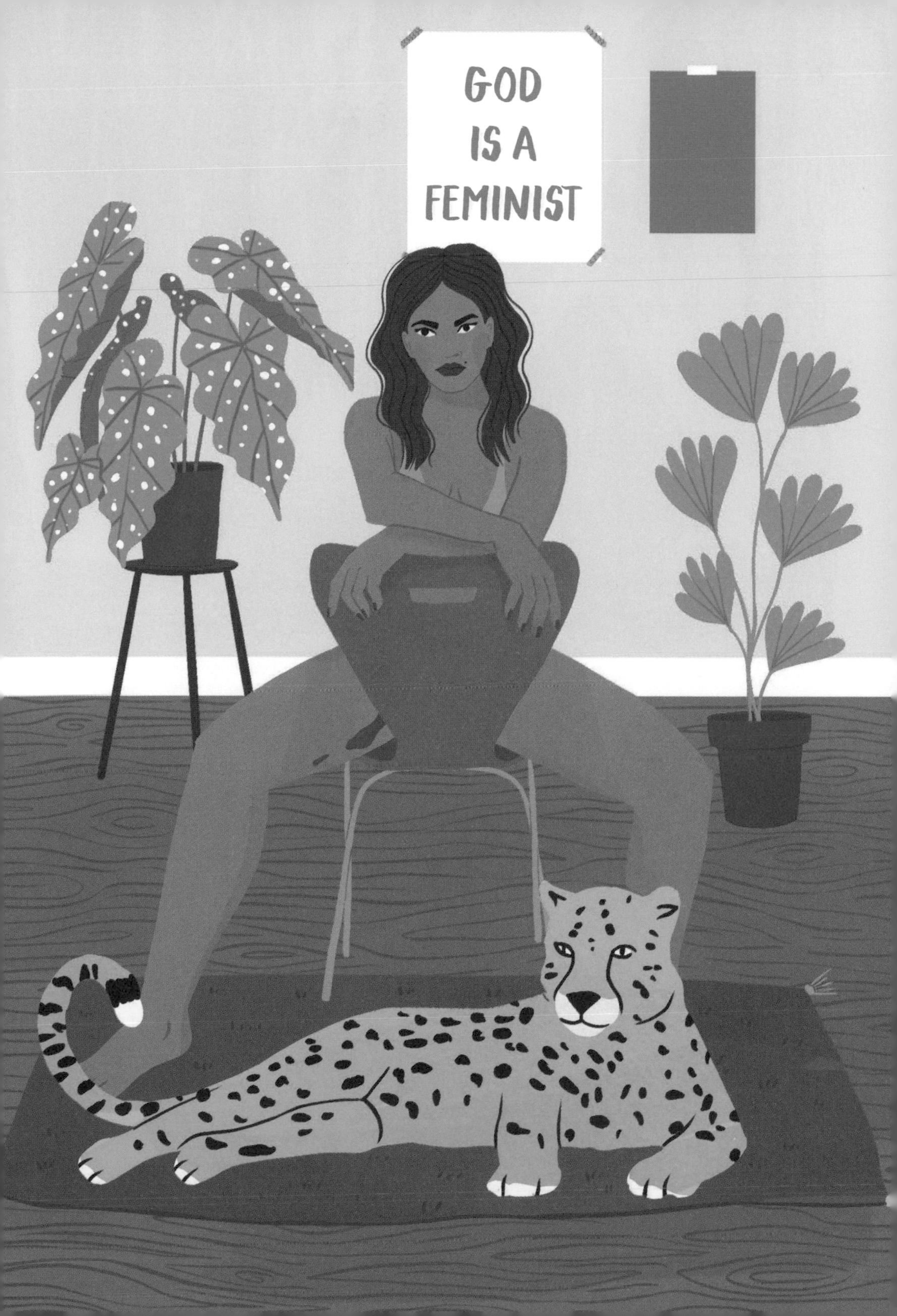
GOD
IS A
FEMINIST

PERIODS ARE NOT HORMONAL

What?! We hate to break it to you but to say 'I'm hormonal' when you are menstruating is actually grammatically and hormonally incorrect. While it is true that, for the week before your period, hormone changes can create premenstrual syndrome, along with a whole heap of physical and emotional symptoms, it is, in fact, the absence of hormones that triggers the uterus to contract and dispel its goddess flow.

So what exactly are these hormones and what are they up to?

Of course you will know that they play a fundamental role in our wellbeing and vice versa, and you now know that many are made in the ovaries. (See page 45, you're welcome!)

But did you know that hormones can be made in the brain? Oh yes! Actually, hormones can be made in almost any organ in the body. You name it, it likely makes a hormone.

'I HATE TO HEAR YOU TALK ABOUT ALL WOMEN AS IF THEY WERE FINE LADIES INSTEAD OF RATIONAL CREATURES. NONE OF US WANT TO BE IN CALM WATERS ALL OUR LIVES.'

Jane Austen

TESTOSTERONE – THE WOMAN'S HORMONE

Repeat after us: 'I am worthy of testosterone.'

You are more than worthy and the whole idea that this is exclusively a male hormone is, well, it's utter nonsense to be frank. Testosterone, produced in your ovaries and adrenal glands, is absolutely vital to a woman's overall health – it helps build bones and prevents bone density loss, plus it supports a healthy balance of lean muscle and fat, maintains sexual vitality and boosts creativity. But how?

Basically, testosterone directly interacts with and is in fact responsible for the release of dopamine, the brain chemical that promotes feelings of happiness. The more dopamine you produce, the more alert, perceptive and attuned to new sensations you are. This is true throughout your life, but in later life, as you go through the menopause, testosterone is paramount for reducing headaches, hot flushes and night sweats, while also helping women to continue to feel energized and invigorated.

MYTH

Progesterone is less important than oestrogen, which is the 'Queen' hormone.

TRUTH

Both progesterone and oestrogen play unique and extremely important roles in your wellbeing. Produced in your adrenal glands and ovaries, progesterone keeps you balanced, can enhance your libido by acting as a precursor to testosterone, boost your energy because it's a precursor to cortisol and support your thyroid hormone, which affects the metabolism of every cell in your body.

Also (yes, there's more!), the monthly release of progesterone after ovulation helps inhibit oestrogen, preventing heavy periods. Progesterone can also help soothe your nervous system, lessen anxiety linked with menopausal hormone fluctuations, and might even be a key player in keeping your skin, nails and hair healthy. Someone pass the progesterone!

MENTAL AND MENSTRUAL HEALTH

There's a strong link between our menstrual cycle and our mental health. You don't say?! But why?

The rise in serotonin, the feel-good brain chemical that enhances feelings of happiness and pleasure, improves mood and decreases feelings of anxiety, plus dopamine (see page 67), alongside oestrogen after menstruation can have a positive effect on our moods and energy levels.

Then, when progesterone comes on the scene after ovulation, it activates GABA (gamma aminobutyric acid), a neurotransmitter, which helps us feel calm and settled.

Normal PMS, before your period, can be a phase where our inner critic comes out to play, making us second-guess ourselves and our choices. For others, it's the time after ovulation, with the highs of progesterone and oestrogen that causes emotional and mental upset.

In the most extreme cases, this could result in a more serious condition called Premenstrual Dysphoric Disorder (PMDD). If it appears similar to normal PMS but with more intense symptoms of irritability, depression, anxiety that turns to rage or excessive crying – sound familiar? Then make an appointment to talk things through with your doctor.

Then there's the mental health impact of the utter fatigue and exhaustion caused by periods, the anxiety connected to the extreme pain of endometriosis and adenomyosis or the burden of waiting years for a proper diagnosis. If you relate to any of this, please know that you don't need to suffer in silence or deal with this on your own. There are so many resources and people out there who can help.

FERTILITY HEALTH IS HEALTH

This can be a hard one to get your head around as our medical system perpetuates the false idea that you only really need to pay attention to your fertility and reproductive health when you have problems with your menstrual cycle or you want to have a baby.

In fact – and perhaps worse – when the medical system refers to women's health it is usually only talking about fertility and reproductive health. Like we don't have any other health?!

Our hormone systems have a major impact on our whole being and should be treated as part of our integrated human health all of the time. If you start to pay deep respect to your hormone system and the changes it brings to your body, not only will you learn what factors might affect the timing of your ovulation – like stress – you will also have a greater understanding of your whole wellbeing; physical, emotional and mental.

CONTRACEPTION

You might think that contraception is a new invention, but birth control has been on the agenda for a while. Today, the most potent question is – why are most birth controls designed to be taken or used by women? Good point. The medical world says – because it's easier to stop a woman's once-a-month ovulation than to block a man's daily onslaught of sperm. We say, 'Nonsense!' We see you, medical patriarchy, and we demand that you now step up.

Either way, we are grateful that we have been given some control over sex without the consequences of a baby. The earliest written record of contraception comes from Ancient Egypt, in 1825 BC, where a papyrus suggested that a doctor apply honey and sodium bicarbonate to the inside of the vagina.

Another early contraceptive technique involved crocodile dung, with conflicting folkloric accounts suggesting that the dung might have been packed against the cervix to block sperm or burned as an incense to ward off pregnancies. Or both?!

In 1870, when the American amateur scientist Charles Goodyear, invented the vulcanization process that enabled the commercial production of rubber, the first condoms were born. Thinner than the crocodile dung at a mere 1mm thick, the first latex condom appeared in 1880.

Almost 100 years later, in 1957, the contraceptive pill was approved – but only for severe menstrual disorders, not as a contraceptive. Low and behold, an unusually large number of women reported severe menstrual disorders. Finally, in 1961 the pill was approved for contraceptive use.

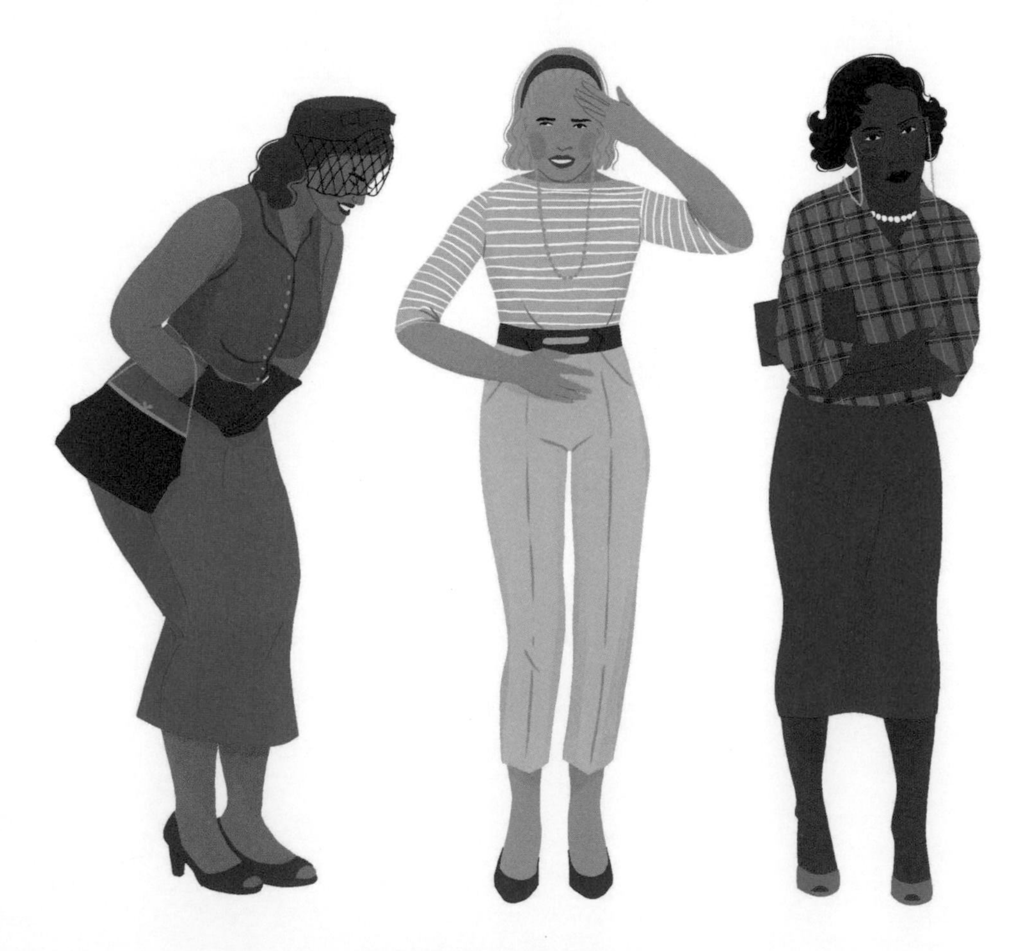

MAKING BABIES & PREGNANCY

Currently in the West, a woman will ovulate approximately 400 times in her life. This number can be deeply impacted by behaviours or health conditions that affect the reproductive hormones, such as anorexia, endometriosis or polycystic ovary syndrome (PCOS), the use of contraceptives which block ovulation and time spent pregnant and breastfeeding. What's really amazing, though, is that in the past, women had fewer periods, inadequate contraception and more frequent pregnancies, historically women would have ovulated less than half as often.

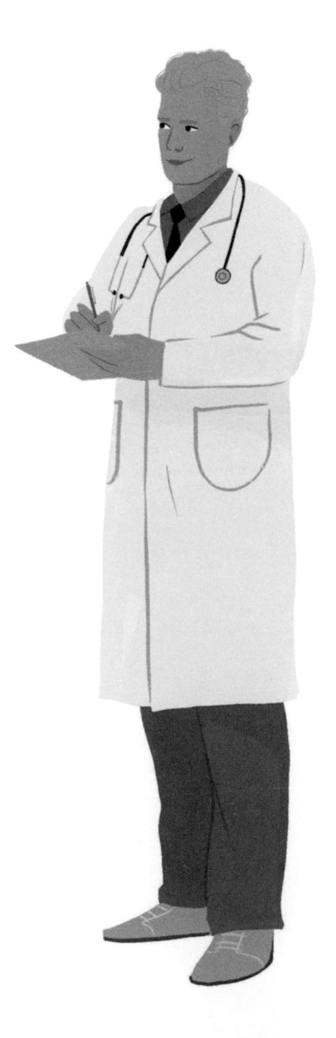

MYTH

Sperm are like an army of sperm that fight their way to the egg, with the fiercest 'solder' winning.

TOTALLY BUSTED

Perhaps our favourite myth ever about women and women's bodies is the idea that the egg is there waiting for an army of sperm to ambush it and fight each other until one finally makes its way through. Recognise this from science class? We thought so.

The truth is that your ovum are unbelievably intelligent and, in fact, invite one sperm to nestle itself into the endometrium and, providing there are no health challenges, create a foetus. Then, once your womb is full, your body will release more hormones during pregnancy than at any other time in your life.

MISCARRIAGE

Miscarriage is the most common reason for losing a baby during pregnancy. About 1 in 10 women will have a miscarriage over a lifetime – a statistic that represents 23 million pregnancies lost annually, or 44 per minute worldwide.

Pregnancy loss is defined differently around the world, but in general a baby who dies before 28 weeks of pregnancy is referred to as a miscarriage, and babies who die at or after 28 weeks are stillbirths. Every year, nearly 2 million babies are stillborn, and many of these deaths are preventable. However, miscarriages and stillbirths are not systematically recorded, even in developed countries, suggesting that the numbers could be even higher.

Around the world, women have varied access to healthcare services, and hospitals and clinics in many countries are very often under-resourced and understaffed. As varied as the experience of losing a baby may be, around the world, stigma, shame and guilt emerge as common themes. Women who lose their babies are made to feel that they should stay silent about their grief, either because miscarriage and stillbirth are still so common, or because they are perceived to be unavoidable.

'AS A WOMAN WHO HAS EXPERIENCED MULTIPLE MISCARRIAGES, THE BEST ADVICE I COULD GIVE ANYONE ABOUT PREGNANCY AND BABIES IS TO STOP ASKING. BECAUSE, IF THAT PERSON IS IN PAIN, IT CAN BE LIKE A MISSILE. STOP ASKING WOMEN WHEN THEY ARE GOING TO GET PREGNANT OR HAVE ANOTHER CHILD. IT'S NONE OF YOUR BUSINESS.'

Myleene Klass on The Happy Vagina Podcast

YOUR CHILDREN DO NOT DEFINE YOU

So, you decided to have children. Amazing! Do you know this means that you are biologically tuned in to your child's high-pitched noises so that you can hear them even when you're asleep?

Yes, that's right – women are incredible. But just as an FYI, this does not mean that your children have to define you. Unless, of course, you want them to – but we would suggest you hang on to YOU for dear life. The greatest lesson you can give your children is to be true to yourself. If they learn this from you, you have given them one of the greatest gifts you can.

'SELF-FORGIVENESS IS EVERYTHING. IT REALLY IS. AND WHENEVER I THINK OF PARENTING, OR WOMAN-ING... I JUST SAY TO MYSELF, PARTICULARLY WITH BEING A MUM, I JUST SAY JUST BE GOOD ENOUGH. THEY HAVE TO SEE THE BALANCE OF THE REAL YOU OR WHAT ARE YOU CREATING? ALL OF THESE DUAL ROLES – INSTEAD OF FIGHTING AGAINST MY SENSITIVITY OR VULNERABILITY, I TRY TO EMBRACE IT.'

Erin O'Connor on The Happy Vagina Podcast

CHILD-FREE

There has been a definitive shift in the last decade, away from the patriarchal assumption that women's primary purpose is to make babies, to a much more inclusive acceptance that women might choose to be child-free for the benefit of her career, the planet, for financial reasons or – and possibly our favourite – it's none of your business.

There are countless reasons as to why you might decide not to have a child. And we are here to tell you – you do not need to have children. And you do not need to explain that to anyone. **THAT IS ALL.**

And if you want them and struggle biologically, there are hundreds of other ways you can do it. From medical support, to being a godparent, surrogacy and adoption.

I THINK STILL IT IS VERY FINE NOT TO WANT CHILDREN. THERE ARE FAR TOO MANY PEOPLE IN THE WORLD. IT'S MY CONTRIBUTION TO ECOLOGY.

HELEN MIRREN

THE DAY OF THE MENOPAUSE

Yes, that is correct, we did say 'the day'. Did you know that, technically, your actual menopause is only one day?
WHAT?! We know!

That is correct. In medical terms, the actual menopause is just one day – the exact day when a woman has not had a period for twelve months. Everything up to then is perimenopause and after is postmenopause.

Postmenopause marks the end of the menstrual cycle, which for many women is incredibly liberating, with no more periods or hormonal headaches and, if you allow it, a much greater sense of reassurance without the monthly upheaval of hormone cycles.

The idea that menopause was a disease was first introduced during the eighteenth century when it was perceived as the worst of all the afflictions. Menopausal woman were seen to have lost their femininity, beauty, fertility and status, and they stood at the gateway to death. These beliefs helped form the basis of modern Western medicine and our attitudes arise directly from such historical perceptions of the menopause.

In the past, people used to say the postmenopausal woman was invisible. We are here to tell you that you are not invisible – you are **INVINCIBLE!** Time to take some risks!

'AT HER FIRST BLEEDING A WOMAN MEETS HER POWER. DURING HER BLEEDING YEARS SHE PRACTISES IT. AT MENOPAUSE SHE BECOMES IT.'
Traditional Native American saying

A SECOND ADOLESCENCE

Not another one? Yes, that's right. The perimenopause can be similar to a second period of adolescence. For most women, perimenopause happens in their forties. These changes in hormone levels may bring irregular periods and night sweats alongside feelings of insanity comparable with your time as a teenager. While you might hope this gives you maximum license to wear heavy black make-up, cry a lot at discos and fixate on pop stars, we would suggest you use it as an opportunity to reconnect and grow into the next powerful stage of life.

There are lots of things you can do to support yourself through this period. Or not do! Swap stress, caffeine, junk foods and late-night discos for more sleep, healthy foods and plenty of exercise. **Heaven!**

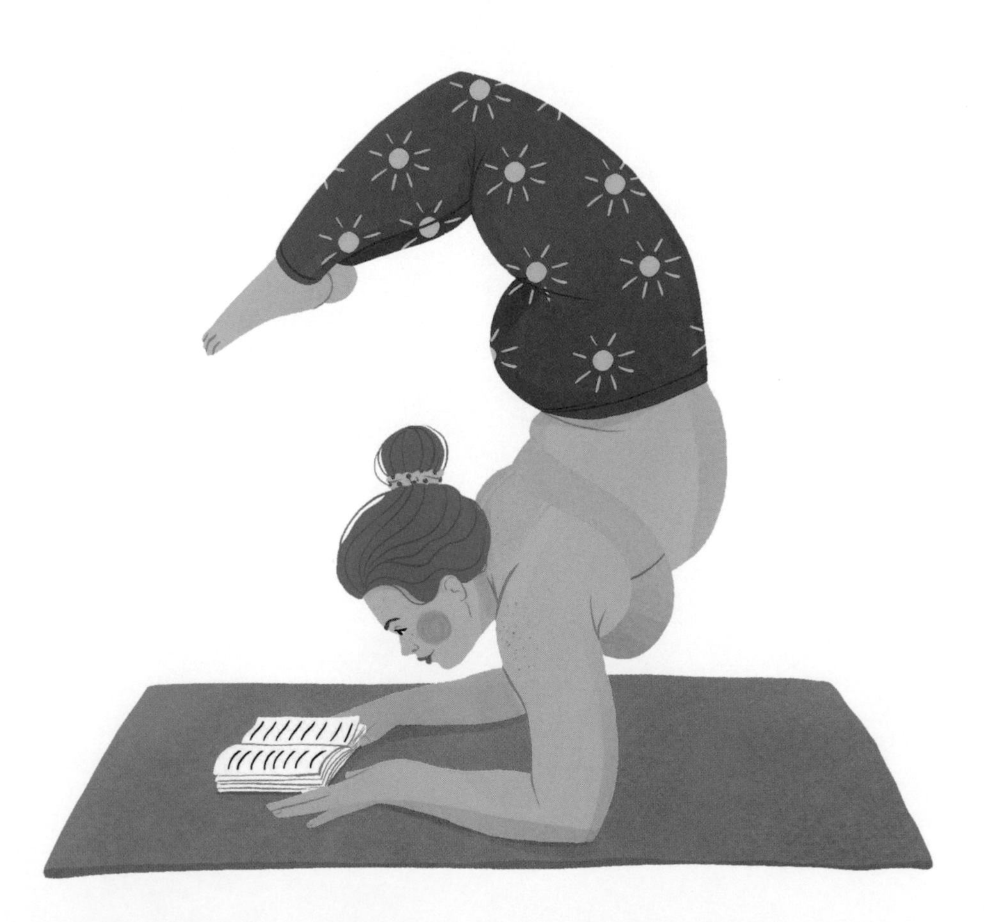

THE GREAT MOISTURIZER

The menopause begins when the levels of oestrogen and progesterone produced by your ovaries drop low enough that you no longer have a regular menstrual cycle. Things like having a hysterectomy or undergoing cancer treatment, such as chemotherapy, can speed up the onset of the menopause.

Made in your ovaries and adrenal glands, oestrogen is a gift – a natural moisturizer that enhances libido, supports connective tissues and keeps the vaginal tissues lubricated. It also works in tandem with serotonin, the feel-good hormone. So, our top tip for the menopause is: moisturize! What, with a lube? Well, yes, that is one way, but then there is bio-identical oestrogen, collagen and masturbation

Masturbation? Yes, that's right – **masturbation.**

Menopause can activate dryness in the vulva and vagina, but the good news is that sex and self-pleasure are proven to increase blood flow to the area. If you're struggling, try some masturbation with an internal sex toy. Menopause campaigners everywhere are reporting that use of a dildo to maintain vaginal resiliency works by training the vaginal muscles to expand and maintain their elasticity. And don't forget a woman's clitoris continues to grow throughout her lifetime, so all of this means that, even with the drop in oestrogen, many women in their forties and fifties can have stronger orgasms than they did during their teens and twenties. You're welcome.

MYTH

Oestrogen is the only hormone I need to worry about in perimenopause.

TRUTH

Oestrogen's effects are closely tied to progesterone. Too much oestrogen without progesterone to balance it creates oestrogen dominance. Why is that a problem? Because increased levels of oestrogen may put you at higher risk of blood clots and stroke. Oestrogen dominance may also increase your chances of thyroid dysfunction with symptoms such as fatigue and weight changes.

CHAPTER 4

THE SEX WAS SO GOOD, EVEN THE NEIGHBOURS HAD A CIGARETTE

LIBIDO LIBERATION

BREAKING NEWS: SEX IS GOOD FOR YOU!

Amongst the many other things missing from the sex education curriculum at school is the fact that sex is good for you. Like, really, **REALLY** good for you. And some even better news: you don't need a partner to reap these benefits – self-pleasure is also part of this equation. So, if sex is so good for us, why don't we have more of it?

Primarily, lack of good education, pain and as per our historical histrionics... shame! Shame about sex overall, shame that we can't achieve climax, shame that we can't help someone else to climax.

Which is all, well, a huge shame!

FRIG

The word 'frig', meaning 'to masturbate', was first recorded in the late sixteenth century, but the word itself was noted at least a hundred years earlier – meaning 'to rub'. It is derived from the latin 'fricare', which also means – you guessed it – 'to rub' and from which also comes the word 'friction'.

TELL HIM I WAS TOO
FUCKING BUSY.
OR VICE VERSA.

DOROTHY PARKER

DESIRE, A RECLAMATION

Throughout history, women have been taught that desire and libido are not for us. It's not so much that it is taught that it is for boys and not for girls, but it is often encouraged in young men as part of the cultural phenomenon frequently described as male bravado. Which, by the way, for some young men is equally as identity damaging.

For young women, the cultural messaging is the opposite. Girls are taught to nurture niceness. To be caring, thoughtful and kind. Pretty much anything outside of this is considered to be a form of overtly sexual acting-out – often called slagging or slutting.

For centuries, a woman's sexuality has been held in this dormant, muted space. Sex was portrayed by religion and experts, including medical professionals, as something exclusively enjoyed by men, while women, in contrast, passively endured it for the purpose of reproduction only. An 1870 advice manual made it clear that girls who masturbated inhibited their glandular development, which would in turn lead to no bosom. **God forbid!**

Thankfully, there is a female sexual revolution happening, right now. Today. Just waiting for you to jump on in!

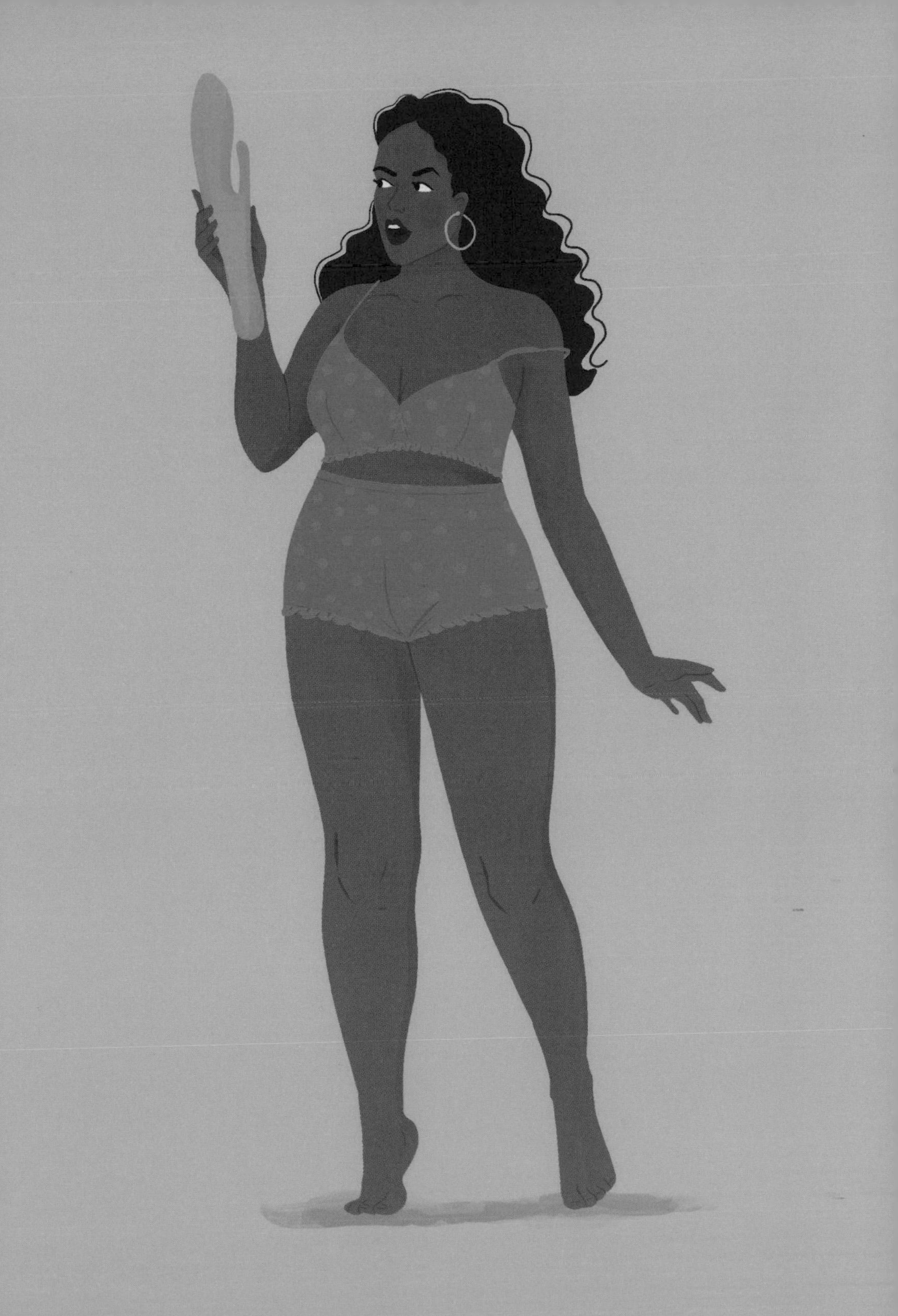

NO SUCH THING AS 'NORMAL'

All this shame, along with a huge dollop of the body self-consciousness culturally ingrained in women, can end up in a lack of libido. But we are here to tell you that not only is sex good for you, but you are entitled to fantastic sex. Yes, entitled. So, let's start at the beginning...

You will have the best sexual experience if you are at your most relaxed and are not worried about what you look like, or about your performance in bed. There is a name for when negative thoughts occur during sex, it is known as 'spectatoring' and it can be a huge barrier to your pleasure. No woman's body, or way to self-pleasure or reaching orgasm is 'normal'. So, the most important thing is to let go of any expectations you may have put on yourself to be this so-called 'normal'.

FUR PIE

A woman's pubic region in its natural, unshaven state. 'Fur' has been used as a slang term for pubic hair since at least the eighteenth century. And to eat fur pie? To perform cunnilingus.

WHY SHOULD WE LOVE SEX? LET'S COUNT THE WAYS...

NATURE'S IMMUNE BOOSTER

Sex increases your immunity, protecting your body against germs, viruses and other intruders.

SEX KEGELS

Good sex is like a workout for your pelvic floor muscles and helps support the uterus, bladder, small intestine and rectum. You can do Kegel exercises, also known as pelvic floor muscle training, just about anytime... And if you reach orgasm, it's a double whammy as it contracts those deep muscles, strengthening them and warding off incontinence.

BOOT CAMP

Sex increases your heart rate and uses various muscles – depending what position you are in – so make sure you mix it up! Like all exercise, it works best when you do it regularly.

DE-STRESS

Touching and hugging enhances oxytocin, one of the body's feel-good hormones, which soothes stress and anxiety. And just like with pleasure, you don't need a partner to reap the benefits. Giving yourself a hug releases oxytocin too. WHAT?! You're welcome!

RELEASE THE PRESSURE

Research suggests a link between sex and lower blood pressure. One landmark study found that sexual intercourse specifically lowered systolic blood pressure.

HORMONAL BALANCE

Regular sex helps keep your oestrogen and testosterone levels in balance.

YOU DO NOT NEED A PARTNER TO HAVE SEX

Listen up: solo sex **IS SEX!**

Sex, pleasure and orgasms are self-care, so we think it's time to smash the taboo around female masturbation, don't you? There's some outdated yet still pervasive cultural stigmatization when it comes to female masturbation and female orgasm. It turns out that getting into a habit of self-pleasure and even, for those who can, bringing yourself to orgasm and experiencing that feel-good dopamine hit and stress relief means that you'll find it easier to experience desire for someone else. Also, because very few women reach orgasm through penetration alone, the better you know yourself, the easier you will find it to teach your partner.

MYTH

Hippocrates suggested that, in order for conception to happen, both the man and the woman needed to orgasm. Galen took this one step further and suggested that a woman would release her own seed at the moment of orgasm.

BUSTED

These wild beliefs were widely held until the nineteenth century when, in 1827, the ovum was discovered. Then, in 1876, Oscar Hertwig identified the fusion of spermatozoa with ova. Today, more research is being done on whether the female climax may have evolved as a mechanism to help sperm move through the vaginal canal and support procreation.

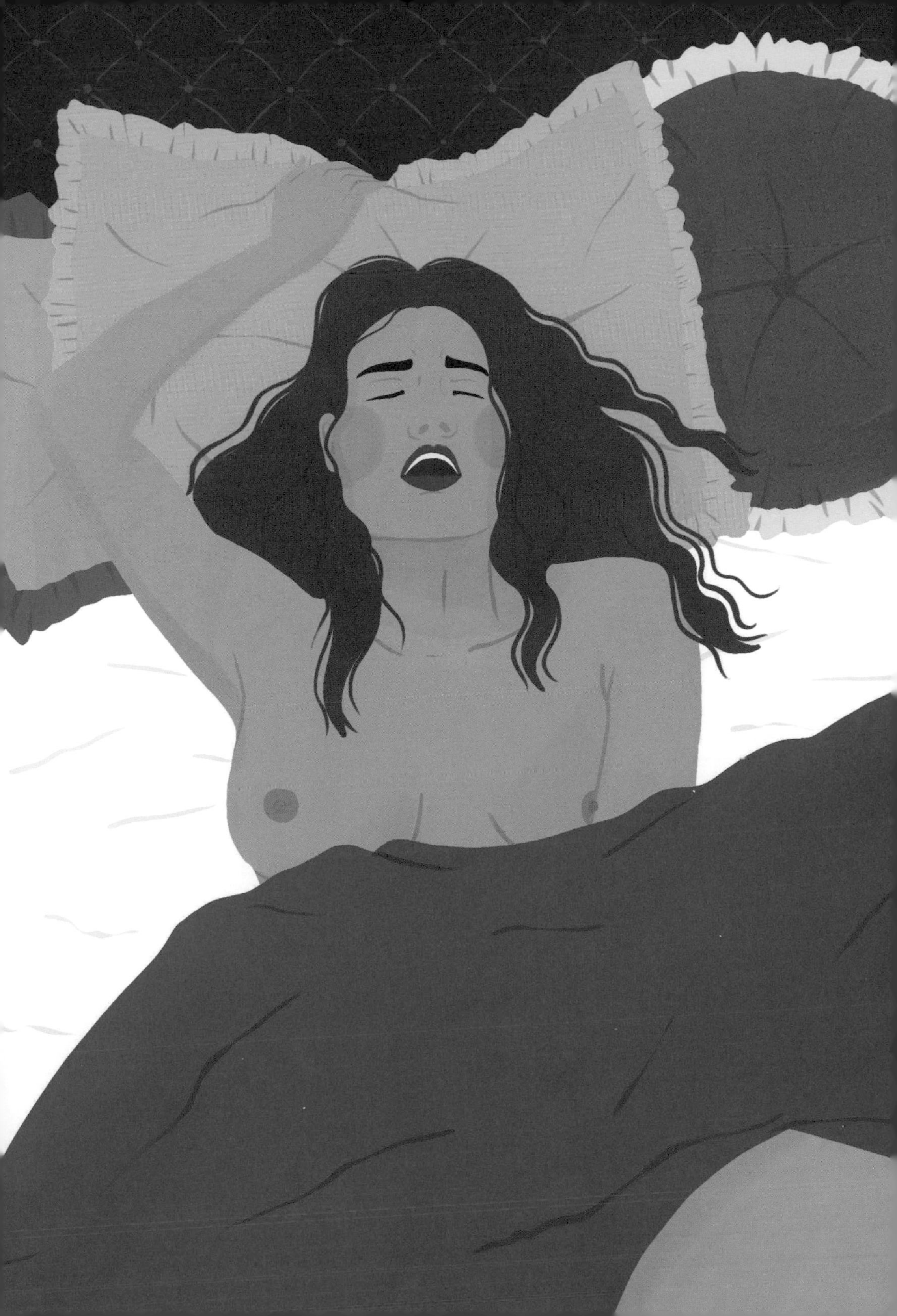

SORRY I'M LATE, I DIDN'T WANT TO COME

Before we get started, let's clear something up – not all women can climax and not all women can climax all of the time. For those of you who haven't yet achieved orgasm, here's a simple deep-dive into all kinds of sexual stimulation, orgasmic or not – you'll realise the benefits are **HUGE!**

GENETICS

We know for a fact that many women aren't able to orgasm, no matter what they do, and it's not because of any inadequacy on their parts or their partner. This is a condition called anorgasmia. It is not a disease or a dysfunction. In fact, research indicates that anorgasmia makes perfect evolutionary sense. Studies suggest a definite link between the inability to have an orgasm and genetics, and according to researchers, it's because those women are evolutionarily choosy about who to orgasm with. In simpler terms, the bodies of some women are designed to not orgasm unless it's with someone ideal to have a baby with.

MINDFUL MASTURBATION

Masturbation techniques used for purpose of easing the mind and re-connecting with your body are becoming more and more popular. These techniques, which do not focus on orgasms, are part of a new trend called 'mindful masturbation'.

One such technique that can promote a healthier state of mind is called 'framing'. Framing is a self-pleasure exercise where you tap into your imagination to reframe the concept of climaxing so it is exclusively tied to ideas of eroticism. It is your brain and your imagination that is most important, rather than touching yourself. Then there is 'edging', which involves you building yourself up to almost-climax, then stopping to rest before starting again. Like self-tantra!

CLIMAXING

As we've mentioned, not everyone can orgasm but that doesn't mean you shouldn't give masturbation a go because there is much pleasure to be had along the journey.

What happens in orgasm? When a woman orgasms, she experiences not just pleasurable and euphoric sensations, but waves of muscles contracting throughout the uterus, as well as the vagina and pelvic floor.

What are the other benefits?

PAIN RELIEF

Before you reach for a painkiller, try an orgasm. Yes, that's right, orgasms can block pain because they release endorphins – chemical messengers in your body that are released by both your central nervous system and your pituitary gland and which play an important part in your body's ability to manage pain and experience pleasure.

For anyone who finds it hard to climax, stimulation without orgasm can also do the trick. Vaginal stimulation can block chronic back and leg pain and, for many women, self-stimulation is an excellent tonic for menstrual cramps, arthritic pain and even headaches.

SLEEP DEEP

You may nod off more quickly after sex, and for good reason. After orgasm, the hormone prolactin is released, which is responsible for post-coital feelings of relaxation and sleepiness.

Finally, as if those two aren't enough of a reason...

DOPED UP

During orgasm, your brain is working overtime to produce a range of different hormones and neurochemicals. One of the key ones is dopamine. Dopamine is the one responsible for feelings of pleasure, desire and motivation.

VIBRATORS

The vibrator was the fifth electrical appliance ever made! Preceding the vacuum cleaner by nine years, the iron by ten and the electric frying pan by more than a decade.

The first electric vibrator came on the market in the nineteenth century and was advertized as good for treating men with pain, headaches, irritability, indigestion and constipation. Sound a bit like hysteria?! It does to us! (See page 19.)

Then, by the early twentieth century, the advertisements started to include women, using the angle of 'for one's health and personal pleasure' and was even featured in advertisements offering cures 'for all disease of the mid-quarters from neck to knee.'

By the 1960s and 1970s, during the sexual revolution, vibrators became portable, colourful and much more complex with so many more settings, sensations and speeds. But it was in 1983, with the invention of The Rabbit, that the vibrator became a self-pleasure staple.

VIBRATORS, THE GREAT TABOO

Vibrators are still taboo in far too many places around the world. And not just taboo – illegal! Did you know you could get arrested for taking your 'bullet' to Dubai or your 'rabbit' to Alabama?!

CUNNILINGUS

Don't know what cunnilingus is? No need to feel ashamed – neither does Siri. We asked Siri: 'Siri, what is cunnilingus?' And Siri replied, 'I don't know what that is.' Shame on you, Apple!

We also asked Alexa and she 'Refused to say'. FFS.

What is cunnilingus? A treasure, that's what.

The word cunnilingus comes from the Latin 'cunnus' which means 'external genitals' and 'lingere' which translates as 'to lick'. So, in a nutshell, cunnilingus means to lick or kiss or suck the lips around the vagina and the clitoris. Yum!

First timer? Before you get down on the going down, let's set the record straight on the vulva. Yours will be different. They all are. In smell, taste, shape, size and colour. You are 100% unique.

YOUR BRAIN ON ORGASM

There is a longstanding theory that orgasm doesn't have anything to do with the genitals at all. Sure, they act as the organs and nerve endings that require stimulation to achieve orgasm, but the actual climax happens only in the brain.

While it will be quite some time before we can confirm this theory or rule it out, some evidence from people suffering from spinal cord injuries does give it credence. Research has shown that women with absolutely no nerve function in their pelvic area due to neurological injuries are still able to orgasm.

TYPES OF ORGASM

> **'EVERY WOMAN IS WIRED DIFFERENTLY. SOME WOMEN'S NERVES BRANCH MORE IN THE VAGINA; OTHER WOMEN'S NERVES BRANCH MORE IN THE CLITORIS. SOME BRANCH A GREAT DEAL IN THE PERINEUM, OR AT THE MOUTH OF THE CERVIX. THAT ACCOUNTS FOR SOME OF THE DIFFERENCES IN FEMALE SEXUAL RESPONSE.'**
>
> Naomi Wolf, *Vagina: A New Biography*

We are finally starting to collectively acknowledge that penis-in-vagina sex alone is rarely, if ever, the key to female orgasms. If you do want to focus on achieving orgasms, here are some things to try:

CLITORAL

A clitoral orgasm results from direct stimulation of the clitoris and surrounding tissue.

G SPOT

We've found ours. Have you? Don't give up! The G spot is actually part of your clitoral network. Let's call it the 'back end'. When you're aroused, your G spot hardens and doubles in size, so let's start there shall we? Trace a line from your belly button to the top of your pubic bone, then insert your finger and press around the area. It's usually more comfortable to seek it out while lying down, or squatting might give you deeper access. If that feels like hard work, grab a G-spot vibrator.

A SPOT

Technically known as the anterior fornix erogenous zone, this pleasure point is located deep inside the vagina between the cervix and the bladder. Also referred to as the female degenerated prostate because of its precise location and ability to be stimulated similarly to the male prostate.

U SPOT

The U spot is another important area that may be easier for some women to find than the A spot. Positioned at the opening of the vagina, directly above and to either side of the urethral opening where women urinate from. Often referred to as the female prostate, the U spot can produce very pleasurable and powerful erotic sensations when stroked lightly. And since it's easier to see, it's easier to find than the mysterious G spot.

V SPOT

Any orgasm you might have that involves exquisite stimulation of the vulva. Oh yes – **Viva La Vulva!!**

VAGINAL

The term vaginal orgasm has been used to describe the orgasm some women have when they are receiving stimulation only from penetration of the vagina.

CERVICAL

Say what? It's true: some women have a cervix that's an actual erogenous zone, and the right kind of strokes and touches during sex can result in an intense orgasm.

SLEEPGASM

The sheer power of the brain means that women can orgasm while they sleep. The female equivalent of a man's wet dream, we've heard that sleeping on your front might help!

NIPPLE

For many women, nipple stimulation activates the same region of the brain as clitoral, vaginal and cervical stimulation.

COREGASM

A what? A coregasm is an orgasm that occurs while performing physical activity like abdominal exercises. Gym, anyone?

BLENDED

We know you aren't meant to have favourites (but THIS is ours!). A blended orgasm is when both a clitoral and vaginal orgasm occur simultaneously, either with the help of a sex toy or a partner. Yes please!

MULTIPLE ORGASMS

If you can have one orgasm, you can probably have another one again, and soon. Once your orgasm is over, your heart rate and breathing return to normal and your vagina and breasts come down from their heightened swollen state. For women, if you want, you can go after another orgasm pretty much immediately.

IT TAKES 237 MUSCLES
TO FAKE AN ORGASM.
BUT ONLY 15 TO SAY
'IT'S A CLITORIS AND
IT'S RIGHT HERE'.

SQUIRTING

Ever felt like you're going to pee yourself when you are about to orgasm? Don't write it off as urine quite yet! In the 1980s, these fluids were scientifically tested and the results revealed a very low amount of urine but a substantial amount of prostate-specific antigen, or PSA.

In men, PSA is produced by the prostate. **HOLD UP** – women's bodies don't have a prostate?! No, not exactly, but they do have prostate tissue in structures known as the Skene's glands or paraurethral glands, which are located on the front wall of the vagina, and some studies show that they drain via ducts into the lower end of the urethra. Research is beginning to suggest that these glands play a crucial part in helping to create the fluids that are released when squirting. Of course, being a 100% uniquely developed human, there are vast differences in the development and size of these glands, which likely explains why only some women experience female ejaculation.

ACTUAL LUBES

When it comes to vaginal lubricants and moisturizers, try to make sure they are as natural as possible; to the extent that they are a concoction you'd be equally as happy to put in your mouth.

If the symptoms of vaginal dryness and discomfort are acute and ongoing, talk to your gynaecologist or a natural practitioner to make sure you are getting the right help, such as a hormone replacement treatment plan if you need one.

DO THESE THINGS TO ENHANCE YOUR SEX LIFE

LUBE UP

The right lubricant can make so-so sex great. There are several types of lube to try, including water- and silicone-based, so experiment to see what works best for you (see page 77).

GET VAGINA FIT

You've probably heard it before, but there are plentiful reasons why you should do your pelvic floor exercises. Why? Because orgasms are your pelvic floor spasming, so if your pelvic floor muscles are strong, your stimulation and climax will be stratospheric!

FISH OIL

Fish oil reduces inflammation, blood pressure and dangerous LDL cholesterol. But guess what? It also raises the testosterone in your body, so you will become aroused more quickly. You can get a hefty dose of fish oil by eating salmon, mackerel, lake trout, sardines or herring twice a week, but you can also use a supplement.

SCHEDULE

Scheduling sex might sound too controlling to be much fun, but sometimes planning is needed in order to prioritize intimacy.

HAVE DIFFICULT CONVERSATIONS

Lost your connection? Communication is lubrication. There is nothing that will ruin a relationship faster than staying mute about your feelings or your desires. Ideally, have the chat outside the bedroom and remember: timing is everything! Then take a deep breath and always start by saying 'I'.

DROP INTO SOME FANTASIES

Getting bored? Do a deep dive into fantasies (see page 100).

DO THESE THINGS TO RUIN YOUR SEX LIFE

FOCUS TOO MUCH ON CLIMAX

Repeat after us: stimulation is as important and beneficial as a climax.

SKIP FOREPLAY

Foreplay is essential to all facets of sexual intercourse. This includes satisfying physical needs as well as the lesser known emotional purpose that helps prepare both parties for sex. It could be both sexual and non-sexual as long as it's done within the context of working towards intimacy. On the mental or psychological level, foreplay is about arousal and preparation. On the physical level, it's important for vaginal lubrication and sexual preparation.

STRESS

Chronic stress may lead to depression and anxiety, and both conditions can get in the way of a healthy sex life.

TOO MUCH ALCOHOL

Alcohol can decrease your vaginal lubrication.

STOP FAKING ORGASMS.

Finally but perhaps most importantly. For the benefit of all genders everywhere – please stop faking orgasms.

While it's OK occasionally to fake pleasure or orgasm, repetition of this will lead to resentment and disconnection. Perhaps more importantly for the wider good, if we fake orgasms, how are men ever going to learn how to stimulate a woman's body?

Some major research needs to be done into why women have a tendency to put their partner's climax before their own, but for now our top tip is – if you are regularly faking orgasms in your relationship, stop. You don't need to make a big song and dance about it, just stop. If you've been lying about how you climax, just tell your partner it's changed. Learn what gives you the greatest pleasure, then teach them.

WHEN HARRY MET SALLY

Way before Netflix's *Sex Education* there was *When Harry Met Sally.* A 1989 romantic comedy written by Nora Ephron where Meg Ryan, as Sally, iconically educates Billy Crystal, as Harry, in the tragic art of fake female orgasm. In a public place. A restaurant to be exact. Her performance is so superb, her fellow diner exclaims, 'I'll have what she's having!'.

LOST YOUR LIBIDO?

First up, don't stress! It's likely nothing to worry about. Libido, or spontaneous sex drive, waxes and wanes depending on many factors. Of course, if what is happening to you is worrying you, then you should consult your doctor and possibly a sex therapist, but in the meantime there are lots of things you can do to help reignite it.

START BY HAVING MORE SEX

Yup, that's right, the more sex you have, the more sex you will want and the better it will be. This is true for all the sexes, but specifically for the females of the species, as having lots of sex increases vaginal lubrication, blood flow and elasticity, all of which make sex feel better and enhance your desire.

BREATHE

Breathing combats stress and connects us to feeling. Breathe deep into your body – all the way down to your pelvis. Your body can hear you – it will respond.

FANTASY

We've established that one of the most important sex organs is the brain (see page 91). So try stocking it with images to reignite your sexual drive.

GET SMELLY

A woman's sense of smell is actually stronger than a man's, especially when she's ovulating. You might find certain smells activate your desire at different stages of your menstrual cycle, so go and explore...

APHRODISIACS

Certain foods, including but not limited to oysters, tomatoes, broccoli and pomegranate juice, are supposed to give your vagina some sparkle.

THE FEMALE GAZE

Anthropologists have found that when people look at a photo of their loved one for 30 seconds or longer, their brain begins producing dopamine, a libido booster. Don't have a loved one? No problem! It turns out that an image of someone you find attractive is just as helpful. You're welcome!

CULTIVATE A FANTASY

In all other aspects of our life, being rational is an asset. But when it comes to the bedroom, let your imagination run riot. Remember, fantasies are healthy and while not every fantasy needs to be acted on (because some may have consequences that could negatively affect your life), exploring them can be a fast track to reigniting a relationship or your own libido.

HOW THOUGH?

First up, get honest with yourself about what your fantasies are. Write them down, visualize them and use that wild imagination. If that seems challenging, check in with yourself and see if you are sitting on some unhelpful judgments and assumptions about different sex acts based on societal norms. These preconceptions often inhibit us from testing out different scenarios (even if it's as a fantasy that only exists in our mind).

Then be brave and share them with your partner. We know it's difficult, but communication is lubrication! Just so you don't feel totally out there, we're here to let you know that the top three fantasies for women are: being pursued (often by a stranger), threesomes and outdoor sex.

GO!

FEMINIST PORNOGRAPHY

There is perhaps nothing that has been more detrimental to sexual relationships between men and women than mainstream pornography with its unrealistic representations of both men's and women's bodies, plus its dogma that women should be merely the recipient of a good pounding.

But we are here to tell you that female-friendly porn can be extremely helpful to expand sexual fantasies with a partner or ourselves. Thankfully, there is now an army of feminist pornmakers who are producing films with realistic representations of women's bodies, stories that align with women's fantasies and – god forbid – fantasy within long-term, loving relationships.

WHOEVER SAID DIAMONDS ARE A GIRL'S BEST FRIEND, NEVER HAD THE RIGHT VIBRATOR.

CARA DELEVINGNE

BDSM

That's bondage, discipline, sadism and masochism to you. Exploring power dynamics with domination and submissive role play can awaken a whole new dimension of your sexuality.

The important thing when exploring BDSM is to develop a strong level of trust and communication. Develop a safe word with your partner, and talk beforehand about what each of you are and aren't OK with trying out.

CONSENT IS A CONVERSATION

This is a huge area and better sex education for everyone is the answer, but just so we are all clear – consent literally means permission for something to happen or agreement to do something.

Did you know in many countries it is illegal to kiss someone who has said 'No'? When someone says 'No' to a sexual activity with you, it means NO.

What's more, consent can also be non-verbal. There are ways to express a clear willingness to engage in sexual contact without using words. Examples of giving non-verbal consent may include nodding their head.

Finally, it's OK to ask again. Feelings, experiences, desire and needs change from moment to moment, so put your ego down and accept the No. And, know you can ask again, in a safe and non-aggressive way, on another occasion.

MONOGAMY AND MARRIAGE

It's OK if you want to get married. It's OK if you don't want to get married. It's OK if you have more than one lover. In fact, marriage and monogamy weren't so popular back in the days of the hunter-gatherers. These communities were nomadic and more egalitarian, giving women a choice of who supported them. This changed with the agricultural revolution when people settled down in one place, requiring a deeper commitment to the family home.

There are, in fact, still societies which operate matriarchal communities. The Mosuo, for example, live on the border of Tibet in the Yunnan and Sichuan provinces. Lineage in these families is traced through the female side of the family and they have 'walking marriages', meaning there is no formal institution of marriage, rather, women choose their partners by walking to the man's home.

This sounds fun to us. You?

SPINSTER

'A woman who is not married, especially a woman who is no longer young and seems unlikely ever to marry'. Um - HELLO?! It's time to reclaim our vocabulary. The word 'spinster' was first used in the thirteenth century to describe women who spun thread and yarn. Tradeswomen who had husbands had access to the markets and better resources (like looms) through their spouses but the women who were not married were forced to take up domestic, low-income jobs like spinning and hence they were called 'spinsters'. Sounds like the first female entrepreneurs to us...

SEX AND YOUR HEALTH

Sexual health includes all of the mental, physical and emotional issues that come with being sexually active. It can impact not only on your relationships but also your psychological wellbeing. Perhaps the most important thing for you to know about sexually transmitted infections (STIs), is that they are NOT something to be ashamed of. The underlying shame about them is in fact not about the disease but about sex itself.

You do need to know that women are more susceptible to STIs than men. **FFS!**

We know. And just for any old-fashioned haters out there – it has NOTHING to do with how many partners you might have had. It's just that women are more vulnerable to infection than men because of the female anatomy being more open, thus making it easier for men to transmit infections to women than vice versa.

You can reduce your risk of getting an STI by using female condoms and insisting that male partners use male condoms.

MYTH

The foot fetish may have developed as a response to widespread STIs.

TRUTH

Yes, you read that right. We did just say foot fetish and sexually transmitted infection in the same sentence. Even if a lot of us may outright deny that it exists in public, foot fetish is perhaps one of the most common types of fetishes around. In a recent study, researchers looked at when the foot was sexualized in popular imagination throughout history. They were surprised to find that all those periods coincided with an STI outbreak in that region, though the study was largely limited to Europe. In a way, it makes sense, as the feet may have emerged as a safer alternative to regular sex when it got too risky.

PHYSICAL PAIN

Discomfort during sex is a very common issue. Physical pain due to sexual activity, such as repetitive penetration, or penetration or friction before the body is fully aroused and the mind isn't turned on, can all be addressed with simple specific massage techniques on the pelvic area and genitals. Sex should feel amazing. If it's painful, physical or emotionally, you need to figure out why. It may be a simple matter of changing positions or adding lubricant. If it continues, please do see a specialist, physical first, then if there is nothing wrong there, a sex therapist could help.

DISASSOCIATION

Numbness can be hard to identify, because not feeling much means that you are likely not to be aware of the numbness. But in the same way that your foot creates a callus to protect it from the damage of rubbing on a new shoe, the skin in our genitals will start desensitizing if we do not pay attention to when something doesn't feel right. Unprocessed emotions and trauma might be one reason we become numb. Or being mute when we are not getting our needs met. Be brave and speak up, and if you need to, take time to re-sensitize your vulva and vagina tissues. Yes, you know it; try some massage and breath into the area to let the nerves know you have heard them and you are responding appropriately.

EVERYONE NEEDS HELP

The longstanding, socially constructed shame we have all experienced about our body and sex means that our mental health and sexual health are inextricably linked. Sexual health is too often thought of in purely clinical terms, like safer sex practices, STIs and contraception. In reality, any of those conversations impact our mental wellbeing and can impact our sense of self-worth. So please ask for help if you need it.

'IT'S THE PLACE WHERE ALL THE MOST PAINFUL THINGS HAVE HAPPENED. BUT IT HAS GIVEN ME INDESCRIBABLE PLEASURE.'

Madonna

CHAPTER 5

BE YOURSELF, EVERYONE ELSE IS TAKEN

FIND YOUR WILD

YOU ARE A GODDESS

By now, we hope you've got the gist of this, but just in case you haven't, we're diving in for one last hurrah, this time out of our pants and into your (potentially) low self-esteem.

It's not that women have ownership of low self-esteem but all the shenanigans noted earlier (from philosophers blowing their own male trumpets, while developing the patriarchy) has certainly left their mark. Women, we believe, are probably the primary victims of this detrimental social conditioning.

Social what? Social conditioning. This is when society trains individuals or a group of individuals within society to respond in a manner that is generally approved of by the society and peer groups within it. All humans are impacted by this but we are calling out to the brave ones – the ones who want to smash the taboos around what it is to be a woman and replace them with the truth about the female organism and **re-find their wild.**

There are hundreds of reasons why all human beings should feel amazing about themselves. So let us share with you some of our favourites about women!

YOU WERE WILD ONCE, DON'T LET THEM TAME YOU.

ISADORA DUNCAN

YOU ARE SPECIAL AND DIFFERENT

YOU CAN BEAR THE PAIN

As we mentioned previously, women can genuinely experience more pain than men. But it's not about strength, it's all to do with memory. Men are more stressed and hypersensitive when they think of pain they've experienced before, while women tend to forget about it faster, leaving them with a pain threshold nine times stronger than men's.

YOU ARE UNIQUELY FLEXIBLE

Yes, every single part of you, and not just your vagina for childbirth, but your whole body. This might leave you with stretch marks and, if you have been blessed with them, we are here to tell you that they are the beautiful. They are your goddess warrior marks that should make you glad you are a woman.

SMALL BUT POWERFUL

Although male brains are larger than female brains, did you know we have the same amount of brain cells? Yup, it's just that the brain cells in a female are simply packed closer together. And it might not come as a surprise to you that the frontal lobe, which is the part of the brain that evaluates options when making a decision, is larger in women than in men.

BRIGHTER IN TECHNICOLOUR

Women can distinguish colours better than men – we literally see more shade. It is also perhaps for this reason that men are more commonly colour blind.

IMMUNITY

Females have higher numbers of and/or higher activity in some types of T cells, which can help trigger adaptive immune responses to viral infections.

COMMUNICATION

Expressing ourselves is something that many (not all) women are exceptional at. And there's even an anatomical explanation for this: women have larger frontal and temporal areas of the cortex, a brain region that is thought to influence language skills.

ENDURANCE

Some studies show that women can perform stamina-related exercise significantly longer than men. The reason for this is hidden in our hormones, as it's thought women's oestrogen makes our muscles more resistant to fatigue.

TO THINE OWN SELF BE TRUE

We hope all of the examples above help show you that you are perfect, just as you are. That does not, however, mean that your life will be perfect, so we also wanted to share with you some suggestions for how to live your very best WOMAN life. Starting with 'to thine own self be true'.

Have you ever heard the expression 'compare and despair'? **OMG.** We know!

Then repeat after us: 'I will not compare myself to others.'

You are not to blame if you have a penchant for thinking this way – we are all at it. It's how our brains are wired within the evolutionary context of survival. Having a cognitive ability to compare our skills with those of others, or to suss out whether or not we might be acceptable to another social group was absolutely essential to our survival tactics. However, in the present day, this type of 'less than' or 'more than' thinking can contribute to anxiety, depression, shame and envy, leading to self-criticism and lack of self-worth, which rapidly undermines anyone's confidence.

SO, HOW DO YOU SHAKE IT?

It's not easy to overcome the habit of comparing ourselves to others and tap into our own, unique, wild self. However, start by taking time each day to be still and meditate on all the things you can be grateful for. Meditation and gratitude go a long way towards combating anxiety and allowing you a more balanced perspective.

But before we lose you at the thought of sitting still for 10 minutes and clearing your mind, did you know that anything can be meditation?! Breadmaking, walking and painting can all be meditation if they allow you some space between your speedy thoughts.

RADICAL SELF-CARE

Beyond the bubble bath, candles and rom-com type of self-care, there is a pioneering, anti-people-pleasing version of self-care that you can access when you decide to put yourself first. This is less about how you look on the outside but more to do with what you need on the inside. The first step to radical self-care is to set boundaries in your life. If you find that hard, don't be hard on yourself. Women are socially conditioned to be people-pleasers, often being made to believe that our role in life is to care, love and organize. Your first step will be to stop caring so much if people like you by getting out of the lane you never wanted to be in, finding **YOUR OWN** lane and then proceeding to win.

YOU ARE TOTALLY UNIQUE

Hang on, haven't you already mentioned that? Affirmative. It was a few pages back (see page 36) when we graced you with the amazing knowledge that your vulva is like a snowflake. Oh yes! And now we are going to bang on about your uniqueness a bit more because symmetry is so overrated.

The more you can embrace your weird and let your unbelievable unique self out, the more your self-esteem will increase.

WONKY BREASTS

Did you know that no woman anywhere, ever, has absolutely symmetrical breasts? And that your left breast is almost definitely bigger than your right? How cool is that? The difference in their size can either be invisible or quite noticeable, and there could be lots of reasons for this. For example, it could be a difference in the volume of breast tissue, the size or shape of the breast pocket, or even the elasticity of the skin on each breast.

ANGER

Anger is a useful emotion and one that women have often been denied due to that aforementioned social conditioning. When you are born with a voice but consistently discouraged from using it, it is not uncommon for this voice to turn on its owner and, in a paradoxical effort to protect, become an internalized critic and source of much psychic angst. Regardless of whether those messages were transmitted by your family or not, they were almost definitely reinforced by society. If you feel angry, there is likely a reason for it. Let it out. Then let it go. Why? Because sitting on a resentment is like drinking poison and expecting the other person to die. Sitting on it will negatively impact both your mental and physical health. Finding forgiveness does not mean that you forget or are pretending that something didn't happen, or even that you have to have that person or people in your life. It is a private experience, inside of yourself, that will enable you to be free, to **stay wild.**

SMASH SHAME

You've heard the expression – you are only as sick as your secrets – right? This is because the things that we keep to ourselves, fearing other humans won't understand, will judge us or, worse, not love us, can become the fulcrum around which negative emotions pivot and, in the worst case scenario, start to impact our life choices. The best self-care love lesson we can do for ourselves is eliminate our shame. Make sure that you have one person in your life you have told absolutely everything to; someone you trust, who champions you and does not judge.

STAY OPEN-MINDED

One of the greatest challenges as we grow into adults is to remain curious and open-minded. Rational and fear-based thinking takes over as we go through life and experience loss and trauma, but a life without judgement will set you free to achieve your goals. Why? Because no one, **NO ONE**, who judges other people is free from judging themselves.

THOUGHTS ARE NOT FACTS

So learn to let go of the unhelpful ones. It's very likely that, in our attempt to persuade you to think about some of your positive qualities, your mind is already coming up with excuses; how some of those good things that you have thought of 'don't count', or someone 'only said that to be kind', 'they didn't mean it', 'they wanted something'... Notice that this is your mind still trying to defend its own prejudice against itself.

WEAR THE DAMN SHORTS

Feeling 'unfeminine', 'unsexy' or 'too large' as a woman is a form of body dysmorphia that has been imposed on us. It grew out of society's need to keep us small. In no uncertain terms, size stigma and dieting is society's modern-day corset, invented to keep us small.

We are not small, or medium, or large. We are women; we come in all shapes and all sizes and we are perfect just as we are. So, fuck diets.

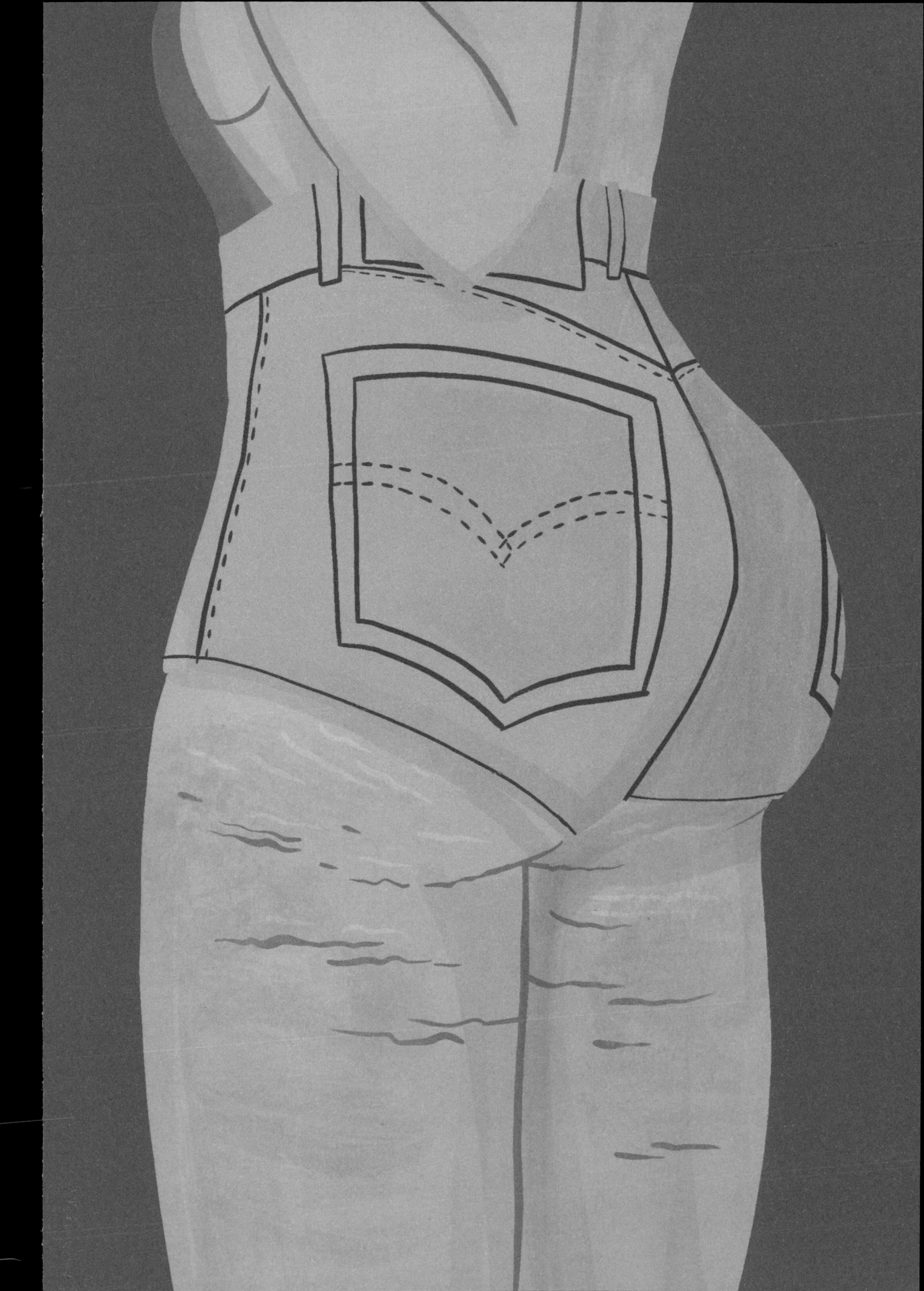

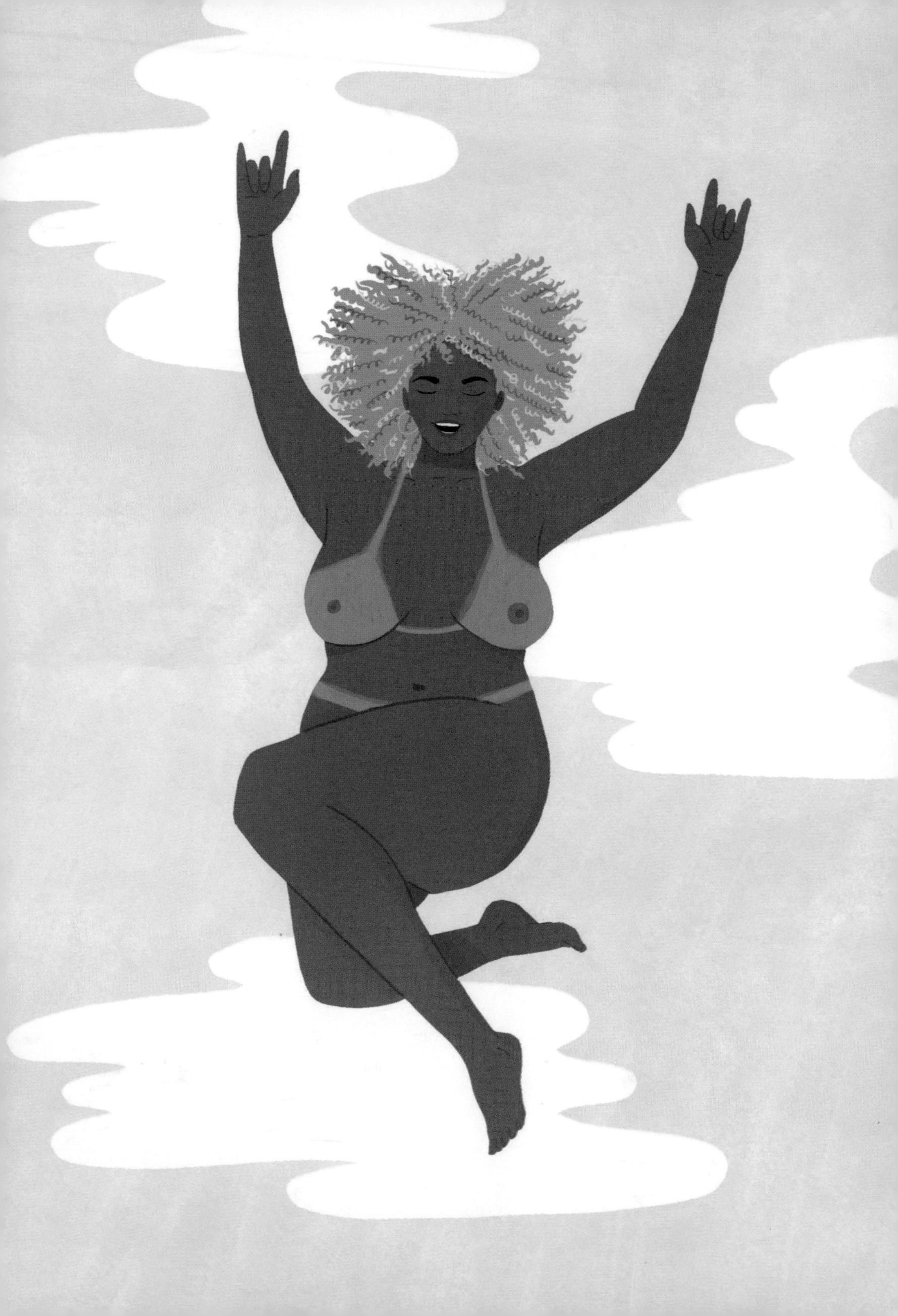

YOU ARE NOT TOO OLD, AND IT IS NOT TOO LATE

Nothing will leave you with deeper resentment than not following your dreams. You will despise, hate and be riddled with jealousy of those who have. 'But I can't,' you say. We say, 'Nonsense'. You can do anything. The real question is: do you really want to?

AGEING IS A PRIVILEGE

Let that sink in.

We spend so much time buying into the myth that the older woman is not valuable, trying to turn back the hands of time on our skin and our bodies. Just pause for a moment and think about what an honour and a deep privilege it is to have the chance to grow old. On average, women live 2–5 years longer than men, a fact which holds true in every country. Why? Well, females are allegedly tougher in utero, our immune systems age slower, we are less likely to take risks that could lead to death or succumb to heart disease later in life, we have stronger social networks and we also generally take better care of our health. QUEENS!

'EVERYBODY HAS A SUPERFICIAL SIDE AND A DEEP SIDE, BUT THIS CULTURE DOESN'T PLACE MUCH VALUE ON DEPTH... WE DON'T HAVE SHAMANS OR SOOTHSAYERS, AND DEPTH ISN'T ENCOURAGED OR UNDERSTOOD. SURROUNDED BY THIS SHALLOW, GLOSSY SOCIETY, WE DEVELOP A SHALLOW SIDE... AND WE BECOME ATTRACTED TO FLUFF... BUT ALONG WITH DEVELOPING MY SUPERFICIAL SIDE, I ALWAYS NURTURED A DEEPER LONGING, SO EVEN WHEN I WAS FALLING INTO THE TRAP OF THAT OTHER KIND OF LOVE, I WAS HIP TO WHAT I WAS DOING.'

Joni Mitchell

RESPECT YOUR ELDERS

If ageing is a privilege, we would suggest you start to nurture a deep-rooted respect for all the women who have led the charge for us since the beginning of time. You might feel like the current personal or global plight is the most important or that your idea for a dramatic change in women's healthcare is groundbreaking, but we can tell you right now, another woman will have paved the way and fought for your freedom so that you can take the conversation further.

You have a duty to learn about the warriors, the leaders and the change makers throughout history. We've added some books at the back to help you on your way! (See page 124.)

BE AN ALLY

You will feel better about yourself if you are. Women are not the only ones who suffer at the hands of patriarchal societies. Allies are people from a group who don't suffer discrimination but who provide support to those who are discriminated against. Allyship, at work in particular, can have many potential benefits: it can foster positive inter-group connections, undermine racism and other forms of oppression and build a more positive social life and workplace culture.

Being an ally is more than being sympathetic towards those who experience discrimination. It is more than simply believing in equality. Being an ally means being willing to act with and for others in pursuit of ending oppression and creating equality.

A LAST WORD ON MEN

All this social conditioning malarkey has deeply affected Western men too. One tragic consequence of gender constructs is that men are 3–4 times more likely to take their own life than women, as seeking help is viewed as a threat to traditional masculinity.

Also, just to rebalance some of our earlier historical histrionics (see page 17), we would like to share with you one titbit from another angle...

Did you know that in sixteenth-century France, women could charge their husbands with impotence as a reason for divorce? The accused husbands would have to prove themselves in a public trial by successfully ejaculating. Nothing is ever black and white, so be kind. Men are glorious, sensitive creatures, desperate for intimacy and to be understood.

ANYONE CAN BE A FEMINIST

'AS FAR AS I AM CONCERNED, BEING ANY GENDER IS A DRAG.'
Patti Smith

You don't need to have hair under your arms, go on demonstrations or hate being wolf whistled at to be a feminist.

At its core, feminism is about independence. About having control over our own bodies. Our own lives. As a movement, it advocates social, political, economic and intellectual equality for women and men. Feminism defines a political perspective; it is distinct from sex or gender. The chances are, if you are reading this book, whatever your gender, you are a feminist.

BE AN ACTIVIST

Doing estimable things builds self-esteem and there is nothing that will help you feel better than supporting a cause or human less fortunate than you. Engage with the issues that you feel passionate about. Here are our top four causes we encourage you to get behind to support women all over the world:

PERIOD POVERTY

Period poverty is defined as having a lack of access to sanitary products due to financial constraints. It is not reserved for developing countries – it is an international crisis. The cost of menstrual products impacts women in any area or household where there is poverty. This is not just a potential health risk – it can also mean girls' education, wellbeing and sometimes entire lives are affected.

Sadly, there's more period poverty now than ever, and a lot of it goes unseen and unspoken about. Despite amazing organizations fighting period poverty, there are still millions of people who aren't able to afford or access the menstrual products they need. This means that it's more important than ever to have a dialogue in our society about period poverty and the reasons it exists, so that we can address it.

If you have the privilege of not experiencing period poverty, we would recommend you support www.freeperiods.org.

OVARIAN CANCER

Ovarian cancer is a type of cancer that begins in the ovaries. It is frequently misdiagnosed and therefore goes undetected until it has already spread to other areas of the body, making it more difficult to treat. Early-stage ovarian cancer, confined to those organs, is easier to treat.

Tragically, the statistics of this disease, which strikes at the most sacred part of a woman's body have barely changed in the past 30 years. Every year worldwide 300,000 women are diagnosed, with one in three of them being diagnosed too late.

While chemotherapy treatments are progressing, there is still no accurate early diagnosis detection test.

For more information and to support medical research into ovarian cancer, go to www.ladygardenfoundation.com.

FGM

What is FGM?

Partial or total removal of external female genitalia. The severest form is known as infibulation, when the vaginal opening is also sewn up, leaving only a small hole for the flow of urine and menstrual blood.

This is a practice that we believe every single woman on the planet should be fighting to abolish. An estimated 140 million girls and women have undergone FGM in 28 African countries, as well as in Yemen, Iraq, Malaysia, Indonesia and among certain ethnic groups in South America and some immigrant communities in the West.

About 3 million girls in Africa are said to be forced to undergo the procedure each year. The cutting is often done without anaesthetic, in conditions that risk potentially fatal infection, often using scissors, razor blades, broken glass and can lids.

Take action against FGM and support www.thefivefoundation.org.

ABORTION

Abortion is an immensely volatile subject, but at The Happy Vagina we believe it should be legal and available for all women, everywhere. But if you don't believe or agree with abortion – don't have one.

Why? Because believe us when we tell you – no woman wants an abortion. However she has ended up with an unwanted, unmanageable pregnancy – whether through rape, failed contraception or lacking the ability to have a conscious thought – no woman actually wants an abortion.

Plus, there is also a vast wealth of information to prove that in the countries where abortion is not legal – women turn to illegal procedures that fundamentally threaten their physical health and often their lives. Women who have assets find a local doctor who will do it privately at cost, or travel elsewhere.

Finally and most importantly, abortion is an international human rights issue. We are incensed that politicians all over the world are using women's bodies to win elections based on the divisive sentiment around abortion. We are incensed that a man, in office, who a woman needing an abortion has never met, can decide on her healthcare, her future. We are incensed that in so many places, in 2021, women are still not being given free choice.

'IF A YOUNG WOMAN WANTS TO HAVE AN ABORTION, THAT'S NO SKIN OFF MY ASS. THAT'S WHY THEY CALL IT CHOICE.'

Jane Roe

If you would like to learn more about abortion, we recommend https://abortionrights.org.uk and https://prochoice.org.

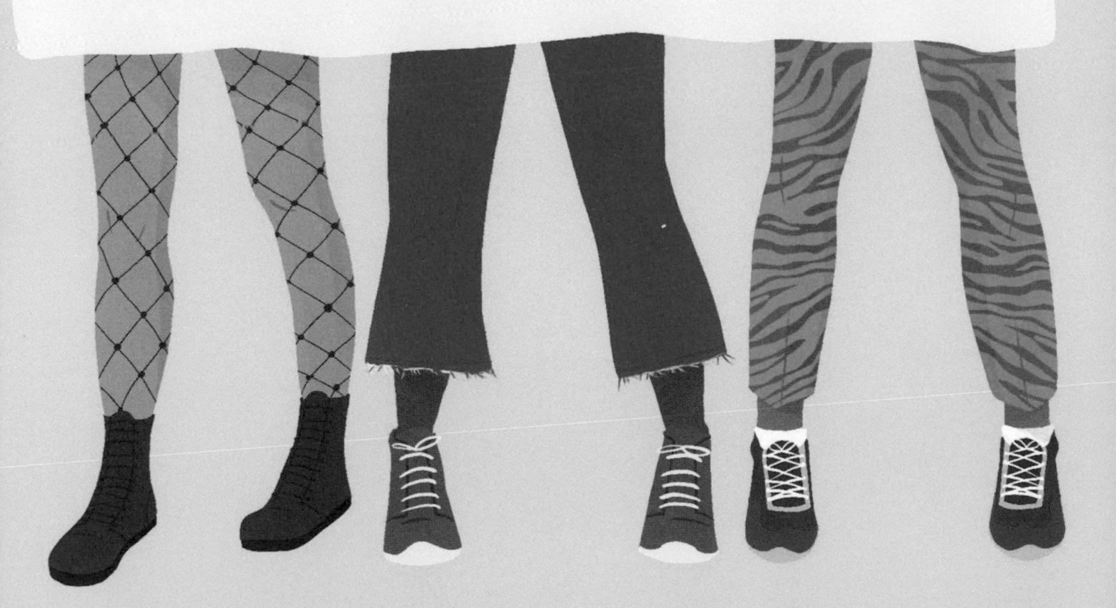
IF I WANTED POLITICS IN MY
VAGINA I'D FUCK A SENATOR

BOOKS TO READ

HEALTH

Period – Emma Barnett
Code Red – Lisa Lister
Unwell Women – Elinor Cleghorn
The Vagina Bible – Dr. Jen Gunter
Raising the Skirt – Catherine Blackledge
Vagina – A re-education – Lynn Enright
Invisible Women – Caroline Criado Perez
Wild Power – Alexandra Pope and Sjanie Hugo Wurlitzer
What We're Told Not to Talk About (But We're Going to Anyway) – Nimco Ali
Read My Lips – Debby Herbenick and Vanessa Schick

SEX

Sex for One – Betty Dodson, PhD
Come As You Are – Emily Nagoski
Girls & Sex – Peggy Orenstein
Sex Ed: A Guide for Adults – Ruby Rare
Nina Hartley's Guide to Total Sex – Nina Hartley
Women's Anatomy of Arousal – Sheri Winston
Better Sex Through Mindfulness – Lori A. Brotto, PhD
Becoming Cliterate – Dr. Laurie Mintz
The Origin of the World: Science and Fiction of the Vagina – Jelto Drenth
The Right to Sex – Amia Srinivasan

SELF-ESTEEM

The Second Sex – Simone de Beauvoir
The Beauty Myth – Naomi Wolf
Difficult Women: A History of Feminism in 11 Fights – Helen Lewis
How to Be a Woman – Caitlin Moran
Revolution from Within – Gloria Steinem
I Feel Bad About My Neck – Nora Ephron
The Vagina Monologues – Eve Ensler
Radical Compassion – Tara Brach
What Would Boudicca Do? – Elizabeth Foley and Beth Coates
The Artist's Way – Julia Cameron
Women Who Run with the Wolves – Clarissa Pinkola Estés
We Should All Be Feminists – Chimamanda Ngozi Adichie

THERE IS ONLY ONE OF YOU IN ALL TIME, THIS EXPRESSION IS UNIQUE. AND IF YOU BLOCK IT, IT WILL NEVER EXIST THROUGH ANY OTHER MEDIUM AND IT WILL BE LOST.

MARTHA GRAHAM

INDEX

A-spot 92
abortion 122
ageing 117–18
Agnodice 26
alcohol 97
allies 118
anasyrma 21, 22–4, 26
Ancient Egypt 50, 69
Ancient Greece 12–14, 18, 22, 26, 39, 48, 64
Anderson, Elizabeth Garrett 27–8
Angelou, Maya 33
anger 113
anorexia 71
anorgasmia 88
anus 34, 35
aphrodisiacs 99
Aretaeus 14
Aristotle 12, 14
Austen, Jane 66

Banks, Elizabeth 63
BDSM 102
Blackledge, Dr Catherine 20
Blackwell, Elizabeth 27, 28
body dysmorphia 114
brain 91, 110
breasts 112

cancer 6, 52, 53, 77, 121
cervical cancer 52, 53
cervical orgasms 93
cervical screening 52
cervix 42
child-free choice 73
childbirth 17, 26, 42
children 73
chlamydia 53
clinical trials 29
clitoral hood 34, 35, 38
clitoral orgasms 39, 92
clitoris 15, 18, 34, 38–9, 77
ClitoUrethroVaginal (CUV) complex 39
colour blindness 110
comparisons 111
condoms 70, 104
contraception 69–70
coregasms 93
cosmetic surgery 36
Crumpler, Rebecca Davis Lee 27
cunnilingus 50, 91

Dalton, Dr Katharina 64
Delevingne, Cara 101
diabetes 53
Diaz, Cameron 48
dildos 18, 77
dissections 15, 16
doctors 19, 51
  women 26–8
dopamine 58, 67, 68, 86, 89, 99
Duncan, Isadora 109

endometriosis 53, 68, 71
endorphins 89

feminism 27, 100, 119
FGM (female genital mutilation) 18, 121
fish oil 96
foot fetishes 104
Freud, Sigmund 39
frig 80

G-spot 32, 39, 92
Galen 14
Gaskin, Ina May 25
gender health gap 19, 29, 32
Graham, Martha 125

Hippocrates 12, 86
hormones 66–7, 69
HPV (human papillomavirus) 52
hymen 40
hysterectomy 77
hysteria 17, 18, 19, 51, 89
  witchcraft 25
immune system 110, 117
India 58

Kapo 24
Kegel exercises 85
Kellogg, John Harvey 18
Klass, Myleene 72

labia 15, 36
labia majora 34, 35, 36
labia minora 34, 35, 36
Leonardo da Vinci 15
life expectancy 117
lubricants 95, 96

Madonna 105
marriage 103
masturbation 18, 77, 80, 82, 86
  mindful 88–9
matriarchal communities 103
medical gaslighting 19
meditation 111
men 119
menopause 38, 44, 45, 67, 75, 77
menstrual cycle 45, 46, 56–68, 76
  changes 58
  curse myth 56
  history 57
  hormones 66–7
  see also periods
mental health 68, 105
merkin 50
mindful masturbation 88–9
Mirren, Helen 74
miscarriage 72
misogyny 12
Mitchell, Joni 117
monogamy 103
mons pubis 34, 35
muff 50

O'Connor, Erin 73
oestrogen 45, 57, 67, 68, 77, 85, 110

open mindedness 114
orgasms 14, 85, 86–95, 97
anorgasmia 88
blended 93
and the brain 91
clitoral 39, 92
different types of 92–3
faking 98
multiple 93
squirting 93
Our Bodies, Our Selves 27
ovarian cancer 6, 121
ovaries 45–6, 67
ovulation 42, 45, 46, 53, 67, 68, 71
oxytocin 85

pain 19, 53, 110
during sex 105
pain relief 89
PAP test 52
paraurethral glands 93
Parker, Dorothy 81
PCOS (polycystic ovary syndrome) 71
pelvic floor exercises 96
pelvic pain 53
perimenopause 75, 76
perineum 34, 35
periods
blood 15, 44
myths about 59, 61
period poverty 120
see also menstrual cycle
pH, vaginal 44
pill, contraceptive 70
placenta 47
PMDD (Premenstrual Dysphoric Disorder) 68
PMS (premenstrual syndrome) 64, 66, 68
popping the cherry 41
pornography 36, 100
pregnancy 42, 44, 47, 71–2
progesterone 45, 67, 68, 76
puberty 45
pubic hair 48–50
pubis 34, 35
pussy 25

quim 52

Roe, Jane 122

Salem hysteria 25
sanitary products 61–2, 120
Sarpong, June 60
self-care 112
serotonin 68, 76
sex
BDSM 102
benefits of 80, 85
consent 102
desire 82
dissociation from 105
enhancing 96
fantasies 96, 100
foreplay 97
loss of libido 99–100
pain during 105
sexual health 104–5
'spectatoring' 84
see also orgasms
shame 113–14
sheela na gigs 22
Sims, James Marion 16
Skene's glands 93
skirt raising 21, 22–4, 26
sleep 89, 93
slut-shaming 41, 42
Soranus of Ephesus 17, 64
sperm 71, 86
spinsters 103
squalene 43
stamina and endurance 110
Steinem, Gloria 12
stillbirths 72
STIs (sexually transmitted infections) 52, 53, 104
stress 57, 97

tampons 44, 61, 62
testosterone 67, 85, 96
thoughts, unhelpful 114

U-spot 92
urethral opening 34, 35
urination 53
uterus (womb) 14, 15, 47

V-spot 92
vagina
anatomy 40
bleeding 53
elasticity of 42
itching 53
opening (introitus) 34, 35
origins of the word 40
using the word 57
vaginal corona 40
vaginal discharge 44, 53
vaginal dryness 95
vaginal orgasms 93
vaginal speculum 16
vaginal steaming 45
Venus of Hohle Fels 21
Vesalius, Andreas 15
vesicovaginal fistula 16
vibrators 89
virginity 41–2
vulva 34–5, 36–9
vulva vestibule 34, 35

water intake 44, 64
When Harry Met Sally 98
witches 24–5
Wolf, Naomi 92
womb (uterus) 14, 15, 47

yoni 43

SPECIAL THANK YOUS

With deepest gratitude to Rosemary Brennan.

Over the ten years I have been working in this field, I have been inspired by the words and writing of many wonderful people, far too many to list. I have brought many of the ideas I have learnt from – and been moved by – together in this book. So really, none of this would have been possible without the wisdom of the incredible community that I am so proud to be a part of. I would like to thank each and every one of you for your constant bravery, intelligence and inspiration.

Special thanks to: Fahren Feingold, Anastasia Achilleos, Chloe Delevingne, Gwyneth Paltrow, Lena Headey, Chloe Macintosh, Dr Zoe Williams, Myleene Klass, Nicola Adams, Imelda May, Dr Susana Banerjee, Aimee Lou Wood, Tanya Reynolds, June Sarpong, Georgia Hirst, Hibo Wardere, Nikita Gill, Meg Mathews, Anäis Gallagher, Andrea McLean, Laura Whitmore, Kate Moyle, Kenny Ethan Jones, Stephanie Yeboah, George Robinson, Emilie Pine, Alix Fox, Charlie Condou, Kate Devlin, Nicholas Pinnock, Jess Megan, Nimco Ali, Erika Lust, Leslie Zemeckis, Ruby Rare, Emily Morse, Dita Von Teese, Alex Light, Erin O'Connor, Paxton Smith, Poppy Jay, Rubina Pabani, Alya Mooro, Nell Hudson, Cassidy Janson, Tara Fitzgerald, Ann Akin, Natalie Campbell, Shareefa J, Sarah Jane Mee, Zoe Hardman, Melissa Hemsley, Millie Hoskins, Rachel Briscoe, Nicola Richardson, Olivia Mervyn-Smith, Amber Huggins, Eleanor Compton, Lola Hylander, Alice Hill, Samantha Brennan, Jessica Mahaffey, Jack Freud, AllBright, Soho House, Epilogue, Rosie Nixon, Bérénice Magistrate, Jackie Annesley, Michael Simmons, Keir Simmons, Jessica Binns, The Brennans, Julia Raffo, Sally Wood, Sally Greene, Berenice Percival, Kate Horne, Chloe Lonsdale, Natasha Pilbrow, Sarah Booth, Dr Stephanie Kuku, Vivien Wong, Amanda Brill, Anabela Chan, Tina Hobley, Miki Haines Sainger, Dr Chandrima Biswas, Teal Cannaday, Amanda Abbington, Julie Graham, Myanna Burring, Tamzin Outhwaite, Kirsty Gallagher, Leanna Best, Ciara Charteris, Maeve Wells, The Scummy Mummies, Julia Rebaudo, Jennifer Grey and my co-founders at Lady Garden Foundation.

All the female centric brands who have given me their time and support – too many to list but you know who you are.

Lastly, but absolutely most importantly, The Happy Vagina community and everyone who has listened to the podcast – without you, none of this would be possible.